The Ethics of Abortion

D0070757

Appealing to reason rather than religious belief, this book is the most comprehensive case against the choice of abortion yet published. *The Ethics of Abortion* critically evaluates all the major grounds for denying fetal personhood, including the views of those who defend not only abortion but also infanticide. It also provides several (non-theological) justifications for the conclusion that all human beings, including those in utero, should be respected as persons. This book also critiques the view that abortion is not wrong even if the human fetus is a person. *The Ethics of Abortion* examines hard cases for those who are pro-life, such as abortion in cases of rape or in order to save the mother's life, as well as hard cases for defenders of abortion, such as sex selection abortion and the rationale for being "personally opposed" but publically supportive of abortion. It concludes with a discussion of whether artificial wombs might end the abortion debate. Answering the arguments of defenders of abortion, this book provides reasoned justification for the view that all intentional abortions are morally wrong and that doctors and nurses who object to abortion should not be forced to act against their consciences.

Dr. Christopher Kaczor is Professor of Philosophy at Loyola Marymount University in Los Angeles.

Routledge Annals of Bioethics

Series Editors:

Mark J. Cherry
St. Edward's University, USA

Ana Smith Iltis
Saint Louis University. USA

The Ethics of Abortion

Women's Rights, Human Life, and the Question of Justice

Christopher Kaczor

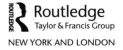 Routledge
Taylor & Francis Group

NEW YORK AND LONDON

First published 2011
by Routledge
711 Third Avenue, New York, NY 10017

Simultaneously published in the UK
by Routledge
2 Park Square, Milton Park, Abingdon, Oxon OX14 4RN

Routledge is an imprint of the Taylor & Francis Group, an informa business

Typeset in by Sabon by Swales & Willis Ltd, Exeter, Devon
Printed and bound in the United States of America on acid-free paper by
Walsworth Publishing Company, Marceline, MO

Library of Congress Cataloging in Publication Data
Kaczor, Christopher Robert, 1969–
   The ethics of abortion : women's rights, human life, and the question of justice /
Christopher Kaczor. — 1st ed.
   p. cm.
   1. Abortion—Moral and ethical aspects.
   2. Abortion—Law and legislation. 3. Women's rights. I. Title.
   HQ767.15.K33 2010
   179.7'6—dc22
   2010018225

ISBN13: 978–0–415–88468–6 (hbk)
ISBN13: 978–0–415–88469–3 (pbk)
ISBN13: 978–0–203–84116–7 (ebk)

Dedicated to
Chad Roper and Jeff Petruska

Contents

Acknowledgments

The first draft of this manuscript was written on a Fulbright Scholarship in Cologne Germany, so thanks is due to the Fulbright Foundation. Thanks also to Jennifer Kaczor, Miles Kessler, Timothy Shanahan, Jason Baher, Dan Speak, Ron Tacelli, Don Marquis, David Solomon, Edward Feser, Frank Beckwith, Michael Pakaluk, Mark Murphy, J. Budziewski, and Peter Vanderschraaf who offered helpful comments on the entire book, or parts of it, at various stages. David Boonin, author of *A Defense of Abortion* (Cambridge University Press, 2003), deserves special recognition and gratitude. David read through the entire manuscript twice, the second time providing me with 23 single spaced pages of comments, questions, objections, and challenges. I am especially indebted to him for this great service.

Portions of the material in this book have appeared earlier as the articles, "The Violinist and Double Effect Reasoning" and "Could Artificial Wombs End the Abortion Debate?" as well as parts of a quarterly column that I write for the *NCBQ*, a bioethics journal. They appear here with permission. I am also grateful for the permission to reprint part of the critique of Boonin's position which appeared earlier in *Life and Learning XVI*, edited by Joseph Koterski. I also represent arguments from chapters two and three of my earlier book entitled *The Edge of Life: Human Dignity and Contemporary Bioethics* (Springer 2005). It seems appropriate to represent, develop, and defend them now against objections appearing more recently. They appear in this book with kind permission of Springer Science and Business Media.

1 Introduction

Teeth clenched, my hands shake slightly. I feel a tremendous surge of adrenaline. I can't believe my eyes. Perhaps the light is not good here, or perhaps I'm holding this little white plastic stick at a bad angle. No. NO. Different lights and different angles lead to the same conclusion. There's no doubt about it, a blue line *definitely* appears where before there was none. The unthinkable, the unplanned, the unwanted is now a concrete reality: pregnancy. What will I do? Who can I tell? What will they say? The questions come too fast to answer.

In various versions, this stark realization takes place every day of every year in every part of the globe. Women differing in race, age, class, and education share center stage in the drama that follows. An unplanned pregnancy can make the women and men involved feel intense anxiety, dread, and shame. Pregnancy can cause great joy, but pregnancy can also cause great fear.

In situations of crisis pregnancy, what could be merely a theoretical debate, pro-life vs. pro-choice, becomes for women and sometimes also the men who made them pregnant a moment of decision, a turning point where life-altering choices are made. Abortion is not, however, simply a concern that faces women with crisis pregnancies. Almost all of us, directly or indirectly, face the issue. Abortion is a subject that confronts health-care providers deciding where to work and what procedures to perform, policy makers shaping social practice, legislators crafting law, voters considering a politician's stand, relief workers seeking to help the poor, and educators teaching health and sex education. Decisions to engage in sex and risk pregnancy are sometimes related to the availability of abortion (Levine, Staiger, Kane, & Zimmerman 1999). Restrictions on abortion for teenagers have been linked to a reduction in rates of teen pregnancy rates and an increase in marriage following pregnancy (Kane & Staiger 1996). The practice of abortion has also been linked to changes in marital norms moving away from "shot-gun" marriage and an increase in single parenthood (Akerlof, Yellen, & Katz 1996). Abortion has also been related to an increase in pregnancy rates, decrease in birth rates, and dramatic declines in rates of adoption (Bitler &

Zavodny 2002). How one thinks about abortion can also be related to how one thinks about other important issues such as stem cell research, euthanasia, and capital punishment. The issue of abortion can even raise deep philosophical questions about what makes life worth living (Spitzer 2000). Abortion uniquely confronts women with crisis pregnancies and the men who made them pregnant, but we all must deal with this issue more or less directly.

This confrontation leads us to raise questions, to be asked and answered, implicitly or explicitly, with great reflection or in a rush to judgment, and various degrees in between. What reproductive rights do women have? Who decides? Is abortion the intentional killing of an innocent human person? Is abortion just the termination of a mass of cells with no more significance than a guppy? Does affirmation of female equality lead to abortion rights? Does personhood begin after birth? Does personhood begin with birth? Does personhood begin with conception? Is abortion permissible even if the fetus is a person?

However, this book will not simply describe various positions taken, pro and con, on these questions but will also critically evaluate them. To proceed as if all views, even contradictory ones, were equally insightful is not to be unbiased, objective, and "neutral." To pretend that all standpoints are equally justified is to take a very strong position, the position of the relativist for whom philosophical dialogue seems pointless, at least as ordered to gaining real insight into what is the case. But such a viewpoint makes superfluous this book or any other book that takes moral issues seriously. Indeed, it makes thinking seriously about anything unimportant, since for the relativist every point of view, however unreflective, prejudiced, or ignorant, is just as "valid" as every other point of view.

1.1 How Should We Talk About Abortion?

Before addressing *how* to talk about abortion, a more basic question is *why* talk about abortion? Almost everyone has his or her mind made up, one way or the other, and so it would seem that there is no use in pursuing the topic further.

This claim is false. Numerous moral issues, once hotly debated, are now objects of widespread consensus, though sadly not practice, throughout most of the Western world. Slavery, women's voting rights, and child labor were once topics of intense political and philosophical dispute, but now a consensus has been clearly reached on each. Likewise, public mores can and have changed radically. Drunk driving was once almost universally tolerated but is now almost universally condemned.

Change is also possible with respect to the abortion issue. Countless individuals have ceased calling themselves pro-life and have begun calling themselves pro-choice, and vice versa. Norma McCovey, better known by the pseudonym "Jane Roe," was granted permission for abortion through the Supreme Court Case *Roe v. Wade*. Not only didn't she get an abortion (the decision was rendered too late), but she now rejects abortion rights entirely, as does Dr. Bernard Nathanson, one of the co-founders of the National Abortion Rights Action League, who had personally overseen some 70,000 abortions, including aborting a fetus he had fathered (Nathanson 1979, 2001). On the other side of the coin, former U.S. President Bill Clinton and Vice President Al Gore were once pro-life, and they now both describe themselves as pro-choice. Not only have numerous individuals changed their minds on this issue and will continue to do so, but each year polls are taken of the general population's opinions on abortion, and each year the polls come out with different results. So long as people have an open mind, about abortion or anything else, it makes sense to talk about the issue.

Such an open approach is essential for the life of the mind. It belongs to human fulfillment to seek insight, perspective, and enlightenment wherever it is found. This implies that upon further examination of the arguments, deeper understanding of the implications, and wider investigation of the evidence, one might change one's mind. In this book, the positions of numerous philosophers are discussed, but one ought not to assume that these philosophers still believe as they once believed. For example, Michael Tooley still defends abortion and infanticide, but his arguments for these conclusions have developed since his early and influential article, "Abortion and Infanticide." Mary Anne Warren likewise shifted her justification for advocating abortion from what amounted to a uni-criterial approach to a multi-criterial approach. Tristram Engelhardt once defended abortion rights but now believes that abortion is morally wrong, on mainly religious rather than secular grounds. I have focused particular attention on those arguments that are either most influential and reprinted (as in the case of Tooley and Warren) or the most up to date and sophisticated (as in the case of David Boonin's *A Defense of Abortion*).

In this book, various shifts in views by authors such as those mentioned already and others will not be traced or emphasized. However, such philosophers provide a wonderful example of how intellectual inquiry should be undertaken—namely with an open mind—open to the possibility of further insight and perspective, even if that enlightenment is in contradiction to what one earlier believed, even if what is actually the case is unpopular with some, and even if that reality is initially hard to believe. One profits most when reading this or any other book in that spirit. After all, the alternative would be to act like the medieval Muslim invaders who came upon the ancient library at Alexandria and were deliberating about what to do with it. As the historically contested account goes, they reasoned as follows. If the books here contradict what is in the Koran, then they should be burned. If the books here contain what is already known in the Koran, then they are superfluous. Since its books are either unneeded or dangerous, the library should be burned. I say this not to recall an embarrassing moment for a particular religious group, for the underlying attitude is found among all peoples. Sadly, a suppression of intellectual curiosity sometimes is found even among those calling themselves philosophers, despite its radical contradiction to the very nature of the human mind as always ordered to further insight.

Although a book like this would have been considered either dangerous or superfluous to these medieval Muslims, the attitude of the reader determines whether the same will be true today. Although almost everyone who reads this book will already have some initial opinion about the topic—whether strongly pro-life, strongly pro-choice, or somewhere in between. I hope that this book is read with a willingness to consider that, just possibly, these initial views could be entirely wrong. After all, entire societies have been quite wrong about various moral matters in the past (e.g., slavery), and it is possible that similar errors might occur again with an entire society or an individual person.

Perhaps the biggest obstacle to thinking clearly about abortion is that virtually everyone knows someone who is strongly pro-life and/or someone who has had an abortion or helped someone obtain an abortion. If we are friends with or are at all sympathetic to such persons, it can be quite difficult to consider the question of abortion carefully. If abortion is *morally permissible*, then our friend or acquaintance who is strongly pro-life would seem to be a deeply misguided and unduly intrusive person. After all, she or he opposes a procedure that is a legitimate exercise of human freedom. In contrast, if abortion is *morally impermissible*, then our friend who has had an abortion or who has helped someone get an abortion would seem to have done something seriously wrong. From the perspective of the pro-life advocate, she or he has killed an innocent human being. If doing what is morally impermissible makes an agent into a morally bad person, it would seem either those who support abortion or those who criticize it are morally bad. Since we cannot easily believe that our friends, neighbors, or family members (or ourselves) are very bad persons, we have a powerful incentive to maintain our present view without much reflection—whatever that view may be.

But this motivation not to judge people as morally evil can easily be maintained without fearing a clear analysis and consideration of the issue. Philosophers have long used distinctions such as that between act and agent, between first order morality and second order morality, or between rightness and goodness. One such distinction is between the subjective culpability of the agent and the objective morality of the act. The objective morality of the act, whether good or evil, does not necessarily imply that the one who discharges the act is good or evil. An act can be ethically impermissible in itself and yet those performing it can be entirely blameless and good. If a brother and sister have sexual intercourse, almost everyone would spontaneously agree that this act is morally wrong. However, if the two were separated at birth and had no idea whatsoever that they were related by blood, on this account the brother and sister would be morally innocent of incest and not bad agents. On the other hand, a person can do a very good act, and yet be a very bad person. Consider a mafia man running for public office who makes a show of his generosity to the poor (in front of cameras, of course) in order to deceive the public about his character. Giving money to those who need it is, in itself, a very good act and yet the mafia don remains a very bad person despite performing it. Indeed, performing this act reinforces his vice, since it proceeds from an evil intention to deceive others who have a legitimate right to the truth.

Judging an agent as good or evil can never be a definitive judgment unless one knows the agent's reason and will. Did the agent fully understand what he or she did? If the agent did not understand, was this ignorance culpable? Did the agent freely do the act or was the agent rendered less than free by intense psychological pressures, use of drugs, or the coercion of others? Since one cannot generally know the answers to such questions, one can have a fixed and firm answer to the question of the morality of the act of abortion and entirely rescind from judging anyone who has opposed abortion or who has had an abortion. One could be 100% committed to a strong pro-choice view, and not judge as evil those who work to oppose abortion. Similarly, one could be 100% committed to a strong pro-life view, and not judge as evil those who have had abortions. Whatever one's view of abortion itself, refraining from making judgments about the character of those touched by abortion (in whatever way) is helpful in treating the topic properly, and more importantly I believe (but won't defend here) that it is an essential part of being a decent human being.

How should this conversation proceed? Some have tried to sway others to their view of abortion by means of religious or theological justification. This work will avoid this approach to the issue by not appealing to theological or religious justifications in the debate. Religion is indeed connected in various ways to the abortion debate, but the links between abortion and religion are not simple and straightforward. There is no clean divide between religious persons who are pro-life and secular people who are pro-choice. Noted religious leaders, including the Rev. Jesse Jackson, support a pro-choice perspective, while distinguished atheistic journalist Nat Hentoff has written in favor of pro-life views. One can make a case for pro-life views using religious justification as Mother Teresa of Calcutta did in her speech at the National Prayer Breakfast, in Washington D.C., on February 3, 1994. On the other hand, one can argue for fetal rights using a secular rationale, as did Bernard Nathanson, writing as an avowed atheist, in his *Aborting America*. One can make a case for pro-choice views using a religious approach, as shown by Dan

Maguire's *Sacred Choices: The Right to Contraception and Abortion in Ten World Religions*. Conversely, one could advocate abortion rights using a secular explanation, as is evident in David Boonin's book, *A Defense of Abortion*. One's religious beliefs (or lack thereof) and one's views on abortion are not always linked in a simple way.

1.2 Loaded Language

This book will attempt to avoid language that needlessly inflames or conceals. Often, those who are pro-choice call their opponents "anti-choice"; those who are pro-life refer to those who favor legalized abortion as "pro-abortion." Both sides bristle at the implications. Pro-life advocates are obviously not opposed to all choices, all liberties, and all freedoms. The object of "choice" is a key factor for determining whether one is opposed to or in favor of any given choice. The most ardent pro-choice advocate is "anti-choice" about any number of things (bombing abortion clinics, withdrawing family planning funding, rape).

On the other side of the coin, even though some philosophers like Mary Anne Warren who favor abortion use the terms "anti-abortion" and "pro-abortion" to characterize these opposing views, but not all who favor legalized abortion on demand personally favor the choice of abortion in all cases or for all people. I am aware of no one writing about this issue who would personally support a late-term, sex-selection abortion against the will of the mother, even if such a procedure is allowed, or even legally required, in some times and places. Generally speaking, for those who favor legalized abortion, abortion itself is not usually understood as good in itself—like feeding the hungry, even when freely chosen; so the label "pro-abortion" they believe is misleading. On the principle that one should be able to name oneself, this book will use neither "anti-choice" nor "pro-abortion" but rather "pro-life" and "pro-choice," terms that appear to be the favored names for those holding the respective views. For variety, I will also use neutral terms such as "defender of abortion" and "critic of abortion."

In addition, loaded language is easily found in speaking about human beings *in utero*. For instance, those that are pro-life point out that "fetus" is a word that dehumanizes human beings in utero and conceals what normal speech reveals. No one attends a "fetus-shower" or speaks of a woman "pregnant with fetus." The clinical term corresponding to fetus for a pregnant woman is *gravida*, but this term is completely unheard of in public discourse. "That *gravida* will give birth any day now." Then again, pro-choice advocates insist that calling the human being in utero "a child" or "an unborn baby" biases the case against them from the start, since only a tiny fraction of the population would assent to killing a "baby" or a "child," even if preborn. I will, therefore, speak usually of the "human fetus," the "human being in utero," or the "fetal human being" as these terms are both scientifically accurate and the least "loaded" towards one perspective or the other.

It should be also acknowledged that, in a biological sense, the humanity of the fetus is acknowledged by those on all sides of the debate. Obviously, those who are pro-life hold that the fetus is human in a genetic sense. But Peter Singer, who is not only pro-choice about abortion but also about infanticide, recognizes the same thing:

> It is possible to give "human being" a precise meaning. We can use it as equivalent to "member of the species *Homo sapiens*." Whether a being is a member of a given species is something that can be determined scientifically, by an examination of the nature of the chromosomes in the cells of living organisms. In this sense, there is no doubt that from the first moments of its existence an embryo conceived from human sperm and eggs is a human being.
>
> (Singer 2000, p. 127)

In this, Singer is not alone. The biological humanity of the fetus is admitted by virtually all informed defenders of abortion as shall be evident throughout this book. So in referring to the human fetus or the human being in utero we do not beg any disputed questions.

Another way in which language can obscure is seen in disputes about the very word "abortion" itself. Those who defend abortion and those who criticize it should be careful to define what is meant by "abortion," both for the sake of clarity and in order to avoid needless arguments, which at bottom are merely semantic rather than substantive. Killing a human being soon after birth is not abortion but infanticide, even if the infant was born following a botched abortion. Killing sperm and/or eggs in order to prevent birth is not abortion but contraception. Although we all have a general idea of what abortion is, how might one define it?

One suggestion is to define abortion as "voluntarily terminating pregnancy." However, the proposed definition conceals the fact that not all abortions are voluntary. Many women undergo involuntary abortions, particularly in China. Involuntary though they are, these surgeries are surely still abortions. The definition fails in another way as well, for "terminating pregnancy" could apply equally well to vaginal birth and cesarean section (which, in an obvious sense, "terminate" or end the pregnancy), as well as to spontaneous miscarriage. In the future, you might be able to "terminate a pregnancy" by removing a human fetus from the uterus at six weeks and placing him or her in an artificial womb to gestate until full term "birth." A wide variety of very different acts fall under the description of "terminating pregnancy." Hence, defining abortion in this way is too broad, too imprecise, and also too convenient. This misleading language hides the reality of abortion as causing death, even if one thinks it only ends the life of a potential person rather than a person with potential. As Ronald Dworkin's book, *Life's Dominion: An Argument About Abortion, Euthanasia, and Individual Freedom*, puts it: "Abortion, which means deliberately killing a developing human embryo . . . [like euthanasia] are both choices for death" (1994, p. 3). Defining abortion as a choice for death does not, as Dworkin's own pro-choice work indicates, beg the question against abortion. But defining abortion in this way does help avoid some likely misunderstandings.

Pro-life advocate Bernard Nathanson, however, disagrees and proposes this definition:

> Abortion is not the killing of the fetus. Rather abortion is the separation of the fetus from the mother . . . [or] the expulsion of the human fetus prematurely, particularly at any time before it is viable or capable of sustaining life.
>
> (Nathanson 1979, pp. 177, 278)

Although this definition of abortion is used sometimes in the medical community, it is certainly too broad. If abortion is merely "the separation of the fetus from the mother," then every cesarean section is also an abortion. If the human fetus does not die, then an abortion properly speaking has not taken place but rather a botched abortion, an attempted abortion, or a failed abortion. The common usage of the verb "abort" indicates as much. If the captain aborted the mission, the mission is over. If the captain tried to abort the mission or failed to abort the mission, the mission may continue. Properly speaking, abortion is intentionally killing the human fetus. Understanding abortion in this way, again, does not beg any questions, for intentional killing is not necessarily wrong as the killing of insects and human beings in self-defense makes clear.

1.3 Women and Abortion

Although the disputes surrounding abortion are manifold and complex, one obvious truth is accepted by the most ardent defenders of abortion as well as by its most ardent critics, namely that women considering abortion are undoubtedly persons. Whether the human fetus merits being protected by law and welcomed in life is a disputed question, but at least in the modern West there is virtually no dispute about the merit and respect due to women. Even though women do not always receive the respect they deserve, and perfect equality between the sexes remains more a goal than a reality, almost no one would publicly call into question the fundamental equality of women as persons with men, and so almost no one denies that women have rights and dignity and therefore always merit consideration and respect.

From the respect due to women, it makes sense to recognize the views and the experiences of women since they are at the center and not at the outskirts of the abortion issue. However, as one might expect, there is simply no such thing as *the* women's perspective on abortion or *the* experience of women with abortion. There is no female perspective on this issue any more than there is a male perspective or a brown-eyed person's perspective. Of course, one could appeal to polls to determine what a majority of women think about abortion. It may be surprising but the polls consistently show that women as a group are less likely to be in favor of abortion than are men. However, such polls have little value for considerations of the moral permissibility of abortion, for at least two reasons. Although polls have some value in determining what people believe to be true, it is also true that the wording of a poll question can and does shape the results. The use of the words "right to choose" or "abortion" can make a significant difference in the numbers of people supporting the procedure. Another reason not to rely on polls in determining moral permissibility is that even if a vast majority of people believe something to be the case, it could turn out that the vast majority of people are mistaken. Polls taken in previous ages would have approved of slavery, wife beating, and child labor, but clearly the majority in these ages made and approved of moral errors, and we have no reason to believe a majority in our age is ethically infallible.

Even among self-described feminists one can find starkly contrasting views of abortion. Susan Sherwin, for example, presents an important summary of what might be called the conventional feminist view of abortion (Sherwin 1996). According to her, abortion is permissible on demand, throughout pregnancy, and without apology. Abortion is a boon for women, and the fetus has no important moral standing. In the *New Republic*, Naomi Wolf offers a nuanced corrective to the conventional feminist view (Wolf 1995). Although she favors abortion rights, Wolf also believes that the conventional feminist account leaves out important elements of the experience of women with abortion and important facts about the human fetus. So, one could perhaps summarize her view in noting that abortion is good for women, though not without qualification, and the human fetus has less value than a woman but is not devoid of value. Finally, Frederica Mathewes-Green (1997), who describes herself as a pro-life feminist, takes Wolf's analysis a step further. Abortion ends the lives of valuable human beings in utero (more than half of them females) and also harms women physically, psychologically, spiritually, and morally. Feminists, let alone women in general, do not share a single view about the abortion issue, either in terms of whether abortion is good for women or about whether the human fetus has moral value.

With respect to the question of whether abortion is good for women *in terms of physical health*, this aspect of the question is strictly empirical and, so, can only be answered via empirical studies. For example, does abortion cause an increased likelihood of breast cancer? Some 28 of 37 studies have shown a link between abortion and breast cancer, but there is still a great deal of debate about the link (for a discussion accessible to the non-specialist, see Hoopes 2002). To what degree does abortion increase the likelihood of future ectopic pregnancy? Is abortion more risky or less risky than giving birth for a woman's health in the short term and in the long term? How likely is it that abortion will lead to reduced future fertility or render a woman permanently sterile? Although both legal and illegal abortions can lead to cervical injury, perforated uterus, or even death, the relative likelihood of such consequences, as well as other health risks, is a matter for empirical determination (for an overview, see Ring-Cassidy & Gentles 2002). These empirical questions must be answered by experts competent in their respective fields and fall outside the scope of ethics. Ethics may make use of the findings of empirical research, or even criticize the methodology of empirical research, but the gathering and collation of such evidence falls outside of an ethical inquiry like this one.

In addition to possible physical well-being, the question of whether abortion is good for women also could be approached in terms of *psychological well-being*. Some women report no adverse effects from their abortions, and some report even feeling freed and exhilarated. Other women report negative experiences and have founded support groups such as Women Exploited by Abortion (WEBA), American Victims of Abortion, and Project Rachael which seek to bring healing and hope to such women. Even some who support legal abortion acknowledge that women can experience severe psychological repercussions following abortion (Torre-Bueno 1997).

Undoubtedly, many women deeply regret their decision to abort, and it would be remiss not to take their testimony and experience seriously. However, not all women who have abortions report such adverse psychological effects. There may also be psychological effects involved in *not* having an abortion. Indeed, many questions can be addressed in considering whether abortion harms or helps women psychologically. Does post-abortion syndrome afflict almost all women following abortion, just some, or only those who are already mentally vulnerable? Are women who report no adverse psychological effects from their abortions really in a form of denial (Reardon 1996, p. 69)? If abortion brings about negative psychological effects, can such effects be reduced or eliminated, and if so, how? It is the task of mental health professionals and psychological researchers to diagnose, assess, and determine the origin of such psychological effects and treat mental health problems related to abortion. Whether or not abortion is good for the psychological health of women, despite being an extremely important and relevant question, is again not the same as the question of ethical permissibility.

1.4 Moral Goodness and Human Flourishing

Moral philosophy or ethics asks questions about what is or is not *morally* permissible, and this is relevant to answering the question of whether abortion benefits or harms women. Experts in the empirical and psychological sciences seek answers to questions about the physical and psychological effects of abortion; philosophers seek answers to the *moral effects* of abortion on women and those who support it. In other words, if abortion is morally permissible, then people seeking justice, moral authenticity, and ethical integration may want to choose abortion or support abortion. If abortion is morally impermissible, then people seeking justice, moral authenticity, and ethical integration will not want to choose abortion or support abortion.

If Aristotle is right that part of human flourishing and authentic happiness includes acting in accord with moral excellence (*arête* in Greek, *virtus* in Latin), then women (and men) have a vested interest in acting in accord with the call of moral excellence. To act in accord with moral excellence is to seek and do what is morally good and avoid what is morally evil. In order to *seek and do* what is morally good and avoid what is morally evil, one must *know* what is morally good (ethically permissible) and morally evil (ethically impermissible).

Other philosophers have come to a similar conclusion by holding that there can be no real human happiness without love—a love that seeks what is good and avoids what is evil for all fellow human persons (Spitzer 2000). Centuries earlier, Socrates expressed a similar insight that it is better to suffer evil than to do evil (Plato 1971). Literature also sometimes reflects these philosophical insights. Fyodor Dostoyevsky's *Crime and Punishment* and Shakespeare's *Macbeth* showed how wrongdoing provides its own punishment. Oscar Wilde vividly depicted the self-inflicted harm suffered by an agent who does wrong in *The Picture of Dorian Grey*. Even though rich, popular, and beautiful, Dorian fails miserably in loving others and even himself properly. Dorian enjoys an eternal summer of good looks, at least exteriorly, but a painting of the young man provides a mirror of his interior life, and so it is the portrait that ages and shows his inner state. The more Dorian does wrong and fails to do what is right, the more the portrait becomes wrinkled, repulsive, and vile, even though in exterior appearance Dorian remains exceptionally good looking. On the outside, Dorian is the picture of beauty, but on the inside—as reflected by his portrait—he becomes more and more deformed, at the end unrecognizably horrid. Wilde's novel teaches a lesson about not just Dorian but about all human agents—we become that which we choose. If we choose the good, the true, and the beautiful, then through the self-shaping power of our own choices we become good, true, and beautiful. By choosing the evil, the false, and the ugly, we paint our own self-portrait in the same repulsive shades.

So if Aristotle's view or Wilde's view as suggested in *The Picture of Dorian Grey* expresses true insight, then properly informing one's conscience, seeking out answers to important ethical questions and then acting according to these answers, is a necessary part of human flourishing and authentic happiness. If abortion is morally permissible, then to have an abortion may contribute to the authentic happiness of the women who choose abortion as well as the women and men who perform abortions or otherwise cooperate in obtaining abortions. If abortion is not morally permissible, then to have an abortion knowingly and willingly does not contribute to but rather undermines the authentic happiness and human flourishing.

Although other arguments have historically been offered, the central contemporary argument about the moral permissibility of abortion turns on the moral status of the human fetus. Even if there are other reasons that have been historically given to suggest that abortion is immoral, the most commonly given reason is that abortion kills a human person. To intentionally kill an innocent person is a paradigm case of an act that is morally impermissible, an act that when knowingly and willingly chosen causes immense moral disfigurement to the agent choosing it and to those who cooperate in it.

I should be clear about my own conclusions on this issue. I believe that sound reasoning informed by a careful and fair examination of the evidence leads to the conclusion that the vast majority of abortions are morally impermissible. If the human being in utero is an innocent person, a being with a right to life, then having an abortion would seem to be wrong, for the right to life of one person entails the duty of others not to intentionally kill him or her.

I should also be clear that in this work I am addressing the question of the *moral permissibility* not the *legality* of abortion. The question of legality is an extremely important one, but in crafting a book of manageable size and scope, I have focused on the ethics of abortion. Thus, when I speak of "rights" in this work, I mean *moral* rights, not *legal* rights, unless the context clearly indicates otherwise. Even leaving aside the legal issues involved, this topic is more than complex enough for a single work. Indeed, a work like this might be seen as a necessary preliminary investigation to tackling various legal questions.

The ethical questions alone are manifold. Is the human fetus a person? When does personhood begin? Even if the human fetus is a person of moral worth, is abortion necessarily wrong? To answer the question "Does abortion harm or help women?" in terms of moral harm or benefit, we must address these moral questions. It is to such important questions that we now turn in the next chapters.

2 Does Personhood Begin After Birth?

One way to defend abortion is to defend infanticide, the intentional killing of a baby after birth. If it can be shown that personhood begins sometime after birth, it will be all the more evident that personhood does not begin prior to birth, and so abortion is not morally wrong. One of the first and most widely disseminated defenses of this view was offered by Michael Tooley's article "Abortion and Infanticide" in which he argues for the moral permissibility of abortion throughout pregnancy and infanticide, up to a week after the child is born. At least among modern philosophers, Tooley broke new ground, but others eventually followed him, lengthening the time for justifiable infanticide to a month after birth (Singer 2000, p. 163) or longer. Singer writes,

> If the fetus does not have the same claim to life as a person, it appears that the newborn baby does not either, and the life of a newborn baby is of less value to it than the life of a pig, a dog, or a chimpanzee is to the nonhuman animal.
>
> (2000, pp. 160–161)

This may sound startling; after all, the killing of an infant is often regarded as among the most heinous crimes a person could commit. However, the fact that society currently condemns infanticide does not mean that society, or at least a large segment of it, cannot change its judgment. Within recent memory, nearly all people in Western society also condemned premarital sex, divorce, and abortion itself. Indeed, the ancient Romans accepted putting unwanted infants to death. Nor are such practices only found in the ancient world. Indeed, even today every year throughout the world, thousands of newborn babies are killed outright or left exposed to die. In contemporary China, many infants are put to death in order to enforce that country's "one child" policy, and since male children are generally seen as more desirable, female babies are more common targets for elimination (Parker 2009).

Western countries are not immune from such practices. In the United States for example each year after their birth about 5000 children are killed, and 95% of these are killed by one or both parents (Alcorn 2000, p. 145). A task force that compiled surveys and statistics for the causes of child abandonment found that often the women who had abandoned their babies were led to do so because they experienced fear, denial, and lack of support. They often believed the offspring would shame their families or they didn't have the resources to support the child, so by way of solution they turned to abandonment or stabbing, smothering, or hitting the baby to death. These same reasons are also often used to justify abortion, so it makes sense for Tooley to treat abortion and infanticide together. Many, in practice, even if outside the scope of the law and conventional morality, have already widened the scope of reproductive choice.

The reasoning offered for the startling conclusion that infanticide (as well as, *a fortiori*, all abortion) is permissible is dense and complicated, but fundamentally rests on a distinction between "persons" possessing rights on the one hand and mere "human beings" not possessing rights on the other. The human fetus as well as the newborn are human beings but not persons, and therefore have no right to life. This chapter explores the reasons offered for infanticide as well as some critical responses to it.

2.1 Persons vs. Human Beings

In common speech, we sometimes use the words "person" and "human being" interchangeably. We might even be tempted to think that all human beings, all members of the biological species *Homo sapiens*, are persons and all persons are human beings. Tooley wants to use terms more precisely than this, and he designates "person" as a moral concept meaning someone who has a serious right to life, that is, a right not to be killed (1972, p. 41). It could turn out then that there are beings who are not human beings, but nevertheless have a right to life. In fact, many people believe that there are categories of non-human persons. For example, some animal rights activists hold that intelligent animals such as dolphins and chimpanzees are persons and many people of faith believe in the existence of non-human persons such as Gabriel and other angels, Lucifer and other demons, and the divine Persons of the Trinity: Father, Son, and Holy Spirit. If an alien like ET were to arrive from another planet, promising peace and presenting plans for human–alien cooperation, such a being, though not human, would be a person, the kind of being with a right to life. For this reason, when encountering fictional beings such as ET, the Iron Giant, or Shrek, we instinctively recoil and believe it is unjust when they are the objects of murderous intent. Tooley observes, therefore, that biology or animal make-up is not essential in determining whether a being has a right to life (1972, p. 51). Now, it may turn out that there are no non-human persons, no space aliens, no deities, no angelic beings, no demons, and therefore, it may be that all persons are human. But just as it doesn't necessarily follow that all humans are men even though all men are humans, so it doesn't necessarily follow that all humans are persons even if all persons are human. Thus, even granting that all persons are human (though how exactly this could be demonstrated is far from clear), another question remains, the question which drives much of the abortion debate and is at the heart of Tooley's article. Are all members of the species *Homo sapiens* also beings deserving of respect and thus of not being intentionally killed?

2.1.1 Not All Human Beings Are Persons

Biologically, it is fairly simple to determine which beings should be scientifically classified as *Homo sapiens* and which ones should not. Human beings have distinctive blood, DNA, and tissue. Even if the untrained eye cannot easily tell the difference, scientists can clearly differentiate a human embryo from a horse embryo, or rabbit embryo. In terms of biological classification, there is no doubt that a human embryo, a human fetus, a human infant, a human toddler, and so on through advanced old age are all various stages of life for a human being. So, although the popular discussion is often couched in terms of a debate about the "humanity" of the fetus or a newborn, from a scientific point of view such questions are definitively answered. If the question is whether a fetus or newborn conceived by human parents is also genetically, biologically, and scientifically to be classified as a member of *Homo sapiens*, a human organism, the answer is beyond serious debate. Both those who call themselves pro-life and those who would call themselves pro-choice agree to at least this. Any being, at whatever stage of maturity, conceived by a human mother and a human father must also be human. Thus, all such fetuses or infants are also indubitably human beings, members of *Homo sapiens* (Purdy and Tooley 1974, p. 140).

However, admitting that what is being killed is a *human* fetus or a *human* infant, does not settle the abortion/infanticide debate in one way or the other, for an important question remains: Are all human beings also persons? Might there be some members of the species *Homo sapiens*, sharing human blood, DNA and so forth with the rest of us, who nevertheless do not possess a right to life? These are not mere rhetorical questions. Several authors including Tooley, Singer, David Boonin, Mary Anne Warren, and many others affirm precisely that the fetus is a biological human being but not a moral person.

Finally, and most importantly, Tooley is anxious to refute what he calls the "conservative" or pro-life position that human personhood begins at the beginning of any human life, normally at conception. Sometimes people have identified this view as the Roman Catholic position, but it is shared by many non-Catholics. Strictly speaking, the position Tooley critiques is not "conservative" in any political sense, for many liberals also have been on the record in favor of pro-life views—the former Democratic Governor of Pennsylvania Bob Casey, Sr., comes to mind as does the liberal, atheist journalist Nat Hentoff. Since very few Western countries strictly enforce a right to life of every human being from conception, the pro-life view is not conservative, if conservatives are understood as those who seek to conserve the status quo.

Tooley holds that difference in biological species is not morally relevant (1972, p. 51). As we saw before, a Martian or angel who is not biologically human might nevertheless be a person. Since a difference in species is morally irrelevant, and since the fetus does not actually function as a person, the importance of the potentiality must be assumed by those who defend the right to life of each human being from conception. Thus, reliance on the "potentiality principle" is a necessary condition of the defense of the right to life (Tooley 1972, p. 56). The reason that human children merit different treatment than youthful apes has nothing to do with any current difference in psychological properties or intellectual abilities. Neither ape nor infant functions as a real, acting, speaking, thinking person. However, the young human being, whether in utero or out, has the potential someday to function as acting, speaking, thinking persons. Thus, according to Tooley, the pro-life viewpoint stands or falls with the potentiality principle.

2.1.2 Potentiality Is Irrelevant

According to Tooley, the potentiality of the fetus or infant to become a person is irrelevant. He seeks to show this irrelevancy by the example of a kitten that is injected with a special serum developed by scientists to enhance and develop super-feline rationality (Tooley 1972, p. 60). This serum can turn any young Boots, Whiskers, or Snowball in your neighborhood into a being as rational as Salem the talking cat from the TV show *Sabrina the Teenage Witch*. Let's imagine such serum is readily available and you also have your three cuddly kittens nearby.

Would you have an obligation to turn Boots, Whiskers, and Snowball into talking cats? It might be quite kind to do so, but you certainly would not be obliged to do so. You have no duty to chase around the entire neighborhood collecting all stray kittens and changing them all into rational cats, even though (after the invention of the serum) all kittens are potentially rational.

To see how the kitten example is relevant to the potentiality of the fetus and newborn, Tooley introduces a distinct consideration which he calls the "symmetry principle." The symmetry principle is, "if it is not seriously wrong to refrain from initiating such a causal process, neither is it seriously wrong to interfere with such a process" (Tooley 1972, p. 58).

Similarly, consider two cases (Rachels 1975). Smith enters the bathroom of his young nephew and drowns the child to get an inheritance. Jones has exactly the same plan, is going into the bathroom to drown the child, but watches with delight as the child hits his head and begins to drown right in front of him. Jones could easily save the child but doesn't lift a finger, and the young nephew drowns. Jones and Smith are equally at fault, even though one did something and the other did nothing. One man performed an act of commission, the other man an act of omission; but there is no important difference between the two.

Similarly, if you do not inject the kitten with special serum, a functioning rational animal, a talking cat, will not come to be. If you have an abortion or destroy a newborn, a functioning rational animal, a human person, will not come to be. Not injecting the kitten is an act of omission—the failure to start a process that will have as its end the existence of a functioning rational animal. Having an abortion or destroying an infant is an act of commission—interrupting a process that will have as its end the existence of a functioning rational animal.

According to the moral symmetry principle, there is no important moral difference between act and omission, between not starting a process and interrupting a process. We certainly do not seem to have an obligation to make all kittens rational, thus we have no obligation to let all human fetuses or all human infants develop into rational animals (Tooley 1972, p. 62). Since the human infant and the human fetus have at best the potential to become functioning adult persons (some of course never make it), the right to life position fails if based on the potentiality principle.

In sum, there is no duty to turn potential rational beings into actually rational beings. Further, there is no moral difference between not starting a process and interrupting a process that is already started (the symmetry principle). So, since there is nothing wrong with not making potentially rational beings (the kittens) into rational beings (Salem), so too there is nothing wrong with interrupting the process whereby a potentially rational being (the fetus or newborn) becomes an actual rational being (the human adult).

2.2 When Does Personhood Begin?

If all these attempts to distinguish mere humans from persons fail, what does Tooley supply in its stead? Tooley arrives at this fundamental principle that an organism has a right to life only if it has a concept of itself as a continuing subject of experiences (1972, p. 62). In support of Tooley, and retrieving a definition of person suggest by John Locke, Singer defines a person as, "a being with awareness of his or her own existence, and the capacity to have wants and plans for the future" (1994, p. 218). This definition of personhood, arising from Locke (1996, p. 138) and amplified by Singer, has several elements: A being is a person if and only if the being has (1) an awareness of his or her own existence (2) over time and in different places with (3) the capacity to have wants and (4) plans for the future.

How do Tooley and Singer arrive at this understanding of personhood? Consider for example the right to property. If Jane has a watch, and Jane gives that watch away to Scott or allows Scott to destroy the watch, then Jane's property rights have not been violated in the least. It would be a violation of her rights if she desired to keep her watch in working order and Scott destroyed her property without her consent or if Scott stole her watch. Such examples indicate the close connection between rights and desires. Our rights therefore arise from our desires, and our rights are not violated if there is not a violation of our desires. If Jane asks Scott to take and destroy the watch, then her rights are not violated in her no longer possessing the watch or in the destruction of the watch, since she has given consent to such actions.

Now Tooley is quick to recognize that there are a few important exceptions to this general rule that we do not violate someone's rights unless we contradict that person's desires. In other words, in these exceptional cases, we may violate another's desires without violating their rights or the person may not have a given desire but they still have a right that we could violate. There are, in particular, three such exceptions to the general account of rights presented by Tooley.

The first exception to the rule that rights arise from desire concerns cases involving emotional disturbance (Tooley 1972, p. 47). We should prevent the teenager who wants to kill himself because his girlfriend broke up with him from doing so, and even though he desires momentarily to die, we do not violate his rights by preventing him from taking his own life. Similarly, those with emotional disturbances of various kinds may desire, temporarily or permanently, to injure themselves and yet we do not violate their rights in keeping them from doing so. Large categories of persons, from drug abusers to those suffering from mental illness, endure grave emotional disturbance but their rights in general, including their right to life, remains.

The second exception to the rule that rights arise from desire is when a previously conscious individual becomes unconscious. Obviously, when we are asleep, our desires are sometimes radically altered. If we are put under anesthesia during an operation, we may have no conscious desires whatsoever. Obviously, however, the slumbering or the anesthetized maintain their right to life. We do not want a view in which personhood comes and goes episodically, so Tooley acknowledges this further exception to the rule.

The third exception to the rule involves individuals whose desires may be distorted by conditioning or indoctrination. Suppose the leaders of a cult have convinced their followers to kill themselves. Were we to come across such cult followers just before they drink the deadly draught, according to Tooley's account, we would be justified in preventing them from carrying out their desires. Cult deprogrammers aid families in recovering their children despite the fact that the children, at least at the beginning of treatment, desire to remain in the cult even at the cost of their own lives. In so helping, such deprogrammers violate no one's rights.

On Tooley's view, rights arise from desires, either distorted desires, as in the three exceptions just described, or non-distorted. Now a being cannot have desires, according to Tooley, unless that being first has a concept of itself as an experiencing subject. So, any being without a concept of itself cannot be a person. Given this understanding of personhood, what follows for the abortion debate?

This question can only be answered by a determination of when a human being is able to have concepts, for obviously without concepts there cannot be a concept of the self. Clearly, however, no human fetus has a concept of himself or herself. However, the same thing holds true for a newborn. Just as no one violates my property rights when taking what I no longer desire to have, so too no wrong is done to a newborn or a human fetus in killing him or her because he or she does not have a concept of himself or herself, has no desire to live, and thus has no rights to violate. Thus, Tooley's argument leads to the conclusion that abortion is permissible throughout all nine months of pregnancy and infanticide is also permissible until the baby has concepts. When does a human child begin to have concepts?

There is some debate about this question. Many philosophers, in both the analytic and continental philosophical traditions, believe that concepts presuppose language, so that one cannot have concepts until language has developed (see, for example, Davidson 1984, p. 157; Malcolm 1977; Stich 1983; Derrida 1973). One could adopt Tooley's view about the relationship between rights, desires, and a concept of the self, and yet reject his belief that one can have concepts prior to having language. If one does this, then one has a new line of demarcation by which to differentiate mere human beings from persons. Since a number of prominent philosophers reject Tooley's account of the relationship of concepts and language but very well may accept his view about the relationship of rights, desires, and a concept of a self, it is important to take this view into account, even though Tooley himself does not hold it.

If this view of the relationship of concepts and language is taken, then the termination of young human beings is permissible until speech develops, which varies rather widely among children but begins on average from approximately nine months of age until two and a half, and for some children even later. On this view, not just infanticide but putting older children to death would then be permissible until the being could use verbal expression. If, and only if, you can say "I have a right to life," do you have a right to life. It happens that some children are deprived of the chance to learn language at all, such as Genie, an American girl found at 13 years of age who, isolated from human contact for years, never learned to speak. On this account, she is not and never was a person. And since she is not a person, her isolation in this fashion could not have violated her rights.

Other philosophers, including Tooley, believe that one could have concepts before acquiring language. This renders the acquisition of personhood by a young human being more difficult to determine. Although the more troubling worry for him is whether we, on his account of personhood, mistreat non-human animals who are in fact persons, Tooley suggests that "where to draw the line" is not so troubling, since in most cases infants would be desired by the parents and their lives chosen for continued existence within the first few days after birth. In most cases, the question of whether to terminate the life of newborn simply does not arise (Tooley 1972, p. 64). In other words, there would in all likelihood be very little problem determining when personhood begins since most parents, not having chosen abortion and infanticide shortly after birth, wouldn't want to eliminate their children later. So, Tooley suggests that the practical moral problem can be handled by choosing a period of time following birth for up to one week, during which time infanticide is permitted (Tooley 1972, p. 64). Singer extends the line, using similar reasoning, until a month after birth (Singer 2000, p. 163).

2.3 Critical Responses to Justifications of Infanticide

Needless to say, not everyone has been convinced that infanticide is acceptable. True, the ancient Romans allowed it, but appealing to the conduct of the ancient Romans to justify a practice is a two-edged sword. Although the ancient Romans did permit abortion and infanticide, they also allowed lethal gladiator fights, brutal slavery, and granted the right to a father to put his *adult* children to death, a right only abolished with the Roman emperor Alexander Severus (d. 235). But historical precedents aside, defenses of infanticide typically rest on several highly controversial presuppositions, one of which is that difference in species is not morally relevant.

2.3.1 Is Species Morally Irrelevant?

If difference of species *were* in fact morally relevant, then the defense of the right to life of newborns and human fetuses would not necessarily need to rely on the potentiality principle. Tooley simply asserts that difference in species is not morally relevant, but this is surely a controversial claim, perhaps more controversial even than his conclusions about abortion and infanticide. There is a good deal of contemporary debate about animal rights, but, nevertheless, most people have powerful intuitions about the following three cases which serve as counter-examples to the claim that differences in species are not morally relevant.

First, there is a moral difference between a hit-and-run involving a squirrel and a hit-and-run accident involving a newborn human being, even if the baby killed were a mentally handicapped and orphaned newborn.

Second, even though many people are vegetarians out of respect for the moral worth of animals, there is still an important difference between eating a hamburger and a Harold burger, even if Harold, due to his mental handicap, was no more intelligent than a cow. A condemnation of cannibalism seems to rest, at least in part, on the idea that difference in species is morally relevant. But, a critic might ask, what if special kinds of cows had all the abilities of a normal adult human being? If members of a certain species take on radically new powers, like "fish" that no longer swim or breathe underwater or "mammals" that have cold blood, then they are no longer the same species as their closely related biological cousins. If special "cows" had the abilities of normal human beings, they would no longer, properly speaking, be cows, and it would be wrong to eat them.

There is a third counter-example to the claim that difference in species is morally irrelevant. Although sexual mores have changed a great deal over the last few decades, it is wrong for human beings to have sexual intercourse with non-human animals. The wrongness of bestiality rests on the idea that difference in species is morally relevant in terms of the permissibility of sexual intercourse. But would it not be equally wrong to have sexual intercourse with a human being who had the level of intelligence of a horse? No, the level of intelligence is not the relevant factor, since we do not object to two horses having sex, but we would object to a horse having sex with a severely mentally handicapped woman, even if the horse and the woman shared the same level of intelligence. Is the wrongness of sex with a horse the exact same wrongness as is involved in sex with a mentally handicapped human being who has the level of intelligence of a horse? No, sex with a mentally handicapped human being who cannot give consent is rape, a different sort of wrong than the wrong of sex between a human being (with or without mental handicap) and a horse. Bestiality is wrong, even if the horse "consents." If hit-and-run or cannibalism or bestiality is wrong simply because difference in species is after all morally relevant (for more, see chapter five), then Tooley's critique of the pro-life position on this point collapses.

On the other hand, if one believes in animal rights in a very strong sense, as articulated for example in the doctrine of *ahimsa* as held in the Indian traditions of Buddhism, Hinduism, and Jainisn, Tooley's conclusion is likewise endangered. If all animals have rights, then younger animals are also beings of moral worth. Not only is the adult bald eagle protected by law in the United States but also the young offspring of adult bald eagles. One could easily accept a very broad endorsement of animal rights for all sentient species and still hold that all human beings, in addition to various other species of animals—all dolphins, all chimps, all primates young and old—should be accorded respect and the right to life. If *all* animals have equal moral status (Taylor 1986), this does not strengthen the case for infanticide and abortion but rather undermines it.

Another argument, this one given by Jeff McMahan's defense of infanticide, against the idea that membership in the human species is a source of moral status is based upon human and non-human combinations across the transgenic spectrum.

> Individuals at one end of the spectrum with only a tiny proportion of human genes are unambiguously chimpanzees; those at the other end with only a tiny proportion of chimpanzee genes are unambiguously human beings. The relevant question is whether the *moral* status of any individual in the spectrum depends on whether it has a sufficiently high proportion of human genes to count as a member of the human species.
>
> (2007, pp. 146–147)

Given the transgenic spectrum example, McMahan believes the defender of human life is faced with a dilemma following from the disjunction that either being a member of the species *Homo sapiens* is a matter of degree or it is not.

One horn of the dilemma follows from the assumption that being a human being is not a matter of degree but rather is an all or nothing category. It is hard to believe that a being mostly composed of chimp genes, but who had the brain of a human being would not be deserving of our respect. Likewise, a being composed mostly of human genes but with a chimp brain would not seem to be worthy of respect as human. Rational functioning rather than the proportion of human genes determines moral status.

On the other hand, if being a human is a matter of degree, reasons McMahan, then defenders of life cannot claim that all persons have an *equal* right to life (the equal wrongness thesis), since all transgenic creatures would not be equally human.

At work here is a presupposition that we need not accept.

> Assume that our working genealogical criterion of species membership is undergirded by a deeper genetic criterion—in other words, that membership in the human species is determined by the possession of a characteristically human genome, which is in fact produced only by the fusion of gametes from human parents.
>
> (McMahan 2007, p. 16)

If creatures of mixed origin are manufactured, then we shall have to debate about whether they should be included in the category of persons. But the debate about such creations need not undermine the moral conviction that all human beings—anyone who arises from human parents—should be accorded equal rights. Indeed, if a species of animal is manufactured with a mix of human and non-human genes (itself morally problematic, see National Academy of Science 2005, p. 55), then the species would have moral rights if the species had a rational nature. We would know the nature of the beings in question by observing how healthy, mature members of the species function. Until we had moral clarity about the nature of transgenic beings, we should treat such creatures as if they had moral rights, on the supposition that we should err on the side of protecting what very well may turn out to be animals of a rational nature.

McMahan's own view runs into problems securing the equality of human persons. McMahan expresses skepticism about the possibility of basing the *equal* moral worth of human persons on properties that are *unequal* among human persons, such as psychological capacities or ethical achievement. McMahan's own defense of infanticide, which relies on the psychological properties granting moral status, ultimately cannot answer why we should treat healthy, mature human adults as moral equals since healthy, mature human adults clearly do not have equal psychological (or ethical) properties. As McMahan himself notes:

> All this leaves me profoundly uncomfortable. It seems virtually unthinkable to abandon our egalitarian commitments, or even to accept that they might be justified only in some indirect way—for example, because it is for the best, all things considered, to treat all people as equals and to inculcate the belief that all are indeed one another's moral equals, even though in reality they are not. Yet the challenges to the equal wrongness thesis, which is a central element of liberal egalitarian morality, support . . . skepticism about the compatibility of our all-or-nothing egalitarian beliefs with the fact that the properties on which our moral status appears to supervene are all matters of degree. It is hard to avoid the sense that our egalitarian commitments rest on distressingly insecure foundations.
>
> (2008, p. 104)

McMahan himself recognizes how "dangerously invidious" it would be, both socially and politically, to publicly deny the fundamental equality of a group of human persons. Yet this denial is implicit in the project of justifying private, lethal choices such as infanticide.

2.3.2 Potentiality and the Symmetry Principle

Tooley writes as if the anti-abortion position rests on the potential of the human fetus to function as a rational animal later in life. However, as we shall consider in chapter five, the most common defenses of fetal human life rely rather on the *actuality* and not the *potentiality* of the human fetus and infant. Let's suppose that, contrary to fact, it were necessary that the potentiality principle be endorsed to support the view that infants and human fetuses enjoy personhood. Suppose further we could inject kittens or colts with a rationality serum and thereby change all injected subjects into the likes of television's talking cat Salem or Mr. Ed. Tooley is surely right that we have no obligation to engender such a transformation. But this does not justify his views on abortion and infanticide.

Here, Tooley fails to recognize an important difference between two kinds of potentiality—passive potentiality and active potentiality (active self-development). If a rationality serum were invented, the kitten or colt would then have a passive potentiality for functioning rationally. If some active force (the serum) comes from the outside via injection, the colt or kitten would then be able to develop itself (active potentiality) into a being that could function rationally. Active potentiality is nothing other than growth or maturation, an active self-development. For example, a sapling has passive potentiality to be carved into the leg of a stool, but actively develops itself to become a mature tree. When applied to the case at hand, the kitten or colt has passive potentiality for rationality, the potential to become a being with active self-development towards rationality. The human fetus, on the other hand, enjoys active self-development towards rational maturity. If functioning rationally is the benchmark of respect, a being actively self-developing towards functional rationality (the human fetus) deserves a greater respect than a being with the passive potential to become a being actively self-developing towards functional rationality (the kitten or colt). So even if a rationality serum existed, it would not follow that killing a kitten would be the moral equivalent of killing a human fetus or newborn.

In order to exclude the importance of potentiality in their defense of infanticide, Nicole Hassoun and Uriah Kriegel appeal to the following example, "Consider, however, what we would say if we found out that oysters could be made conscious upon being transported to Mars. This would probably not convince most of us to stop eating oysters on Earth" (2008, p. 51). Of course, a normal human infant develops towards consciousness in the absence of special intervention, unlike the oysters transported to Mars, so Hassoun and Kriegel develop their example further:

> Suppose that many years from now, a space elevator is installed between Earth and Mars, and that an oyster finds its way to the elevator. At this point, the normal course of events should lead to that oyster's becoming conscious *in the absence of intervention.*

The oyster on the elevator is thus potentially conscious in the sense in which foetuses and neonates are—it is, so to speak, *en route* to consciousness. Yet it still seems intuitively permissible to kill the oyster.

(Hassoun and Kriegel 2008, p. 51)

It is difficult to take such a preposterous example seriously rather than laugh and say, "Come on, do you *really* think that killing a newborn baby is like killing an oyster that could become conscious by taking a space elevator to Mars?" The more ridiculous the example, the less useful it is in clarifying real cases at hand. However, if *per impossibile* oysters were indeed immature rational creatures simply in need of the right developmental conditions in order to flourish and exhibit their rational natures, then they would have rights to live. But they are not, and they don't.

In his defense of infanticide, McMahan offers a more powerful critique of the rational potentiality as a source of the value of a human being. He notes that congenitally severely disabled human beings do not in fact have the capacity for rationality. Such human beings may grow to adult size, but they are never able to exercise rational capacities of any kind. The potential for rationality is not, therefore, present in all members of the human species, so the potential for rationality cannot justify the claim that all members of the human species have moral worth as persons. How might one respond?

The ethical realm concerns decisions that promote or thwart the flourishing of various kinds of beings. The importance of species membership is due to the way in which being a certain kind of being is related to distinctive ways of flourishing (Anderson 2004; Nussbaum 2004). For example, if a human being cannot read at the age of ten, then that human being is not fully flourishing; whereas a cat can flourish *qua* cat without reading, and so even if *per impossibile* we could teach a cat to read, we would be under no obligation to do so. Since flourishing is related to species, the natural kind of a being should inform how one treats the being ethically. Human mental handicaps are a painful lack of flourishing precisely because the distinctive form of flourishing of human beings involves the use of rationality. A mentally handicapped girl and a dog may be equally incapable of exercising distinctly autonomous reason and choice. However, this condition is a tragic disability for the girl but inconsequential for the dog. The dog can enjoy his species-specific form of canine flourishing; the girl cannot flourish in a distinctly human kind of way. For this reason, to make heroic efforts to help the girl develop towards human autonomy and choice by removing obstacles to her active self-development as a human being differs morally from similar efforts on behalf of the dog. The moral importance of species membership will be explored at greater length in chapter five.

Even if the difference between passive potentiality and active self-development were not important, the symmetry principle is still problematic. Specifically, it does not seem to be the case that failing to initiate a causal process (not injecting Fluffy) is the same as interrupting a causal process already in process (killing the preborn or newborn human being on the road to functional rationality). The symmetry principle, recall, brings one to the conclusion that if we have no obligation to make the kittens rational animals, then we do no wrong by stopping young humans from becoming functioning rational animals.

The symmetry principle is not self-evidently true. There is sometimes an important difference between not initiating a process and interrupting a process already in motion. Although one normally does no wrong by not making a promise, one does do wrong in breaking a promise one is in the process of carrying out. There is normally no obligation to help a friend move, but if I am in the middle of helping you carry your grand piano up the stairs to the fourth floor and in the middle of the third flight of stairs suddenly decide to go for ice cream, leaving you struggling with the massive instrument, then I've done something wrong. The symmetry principle does not appear to be true because there is a difference between not making a promise and breaking a promise partially carried out.

There is also a morally relevant distinction ignored by Tooley between refraining from making someone better off and acting so as to make him positively worse off. If I refrain from giving you the five dollars in my wallet, I've refrained from making you better off, but I haven't thereby worsened your situation. I've just left you in the same shape you would have been in anyway if I hadn't even existed at all. But if I take *your* five dollars, I've positively worsened your condition, which is obviously morally blameworthy. Similarly, if I refrain from giving the cats the serum, all I've done is left them in just the condition they were already in anyway and were set to remain in and so I haven't left them worse off. To abort a human fetus or kill a newborn, however, is positively to make the human fetus or the newborn worse off, since killing deprives the being of its life (for more, on this debated matter, see section 7.8).

What sense can we make of the Jones/Smith example? Assuming the same motivation and proximate intention, if action A and refraining from action B both result in C, then A and B are morally equivalent. Jones and Smith have the same motivation (the inheritance), and they both intend the death of the nephew (Jones by the act of drowning, Smith by omitting an obligation to save innocent life when easily possible). Jones and Smith both perform evil actions, but they do not perform the same kind of action. Jones murders; Smith grossly fails in his duty to save. How does this relate to injecting potentially rational kittens and aborting human fetuses?

Unlike the duty to save innocent human life when easily possible, it does not seem to be the case that one must create rational beings whenever possible or even when easily possible. Although some philosophers (Grisez 1964; Anscombe 1965, 1975; Finnis 1991; Smith 1991) argue that there is a duty not to render sexual acts infertile by contraception, no one believes that whenever one can create a rational animal, one must always at least try to do so. This view would require every woman to have as many children as biologically possible (more than 20 children for some women) and would require every man to attempt to impregnate a woman whenever conception is possible. Such a duty would probably justify adultery, rape, and incest given likely conception. So unlike Jones who fails to discharge his duty in this situation to save the innocent life of his rich nephew, there is no corresponding duty to make kittens rational animals even if possible. The symmetry principle, even if it were true, would not apply to infanticide or abortion.

2.3.3 Curious Exceptions to the Rule

In addition, some might want to critique Tooley's exceptions to the general principle that rights arise from desires. For example, with respect to the third exception, that one may act against another's desires if these desires arise from indoctrination or brainwashing, Patrick Lee has drawn a parallel between this situation and abortion insofar as killing a fetus or a newborn destroys not only their actual existence but the natural desires that they would have had (Lee 1996, pp. 21–22). Further, as Lee points out, the three apparently *ad hoc* exceptions Tooley makes to his rule might lead one to ask: Why shouldn't cases involving human fetuses and infants also be exceptions? It would seem that Tooley has crafted a rule to include and exclude those that on other grounds he wishes to include or exclude, but then the rule itself is not really the rational ground but only a rationalization. (For the record, Tooley later rejected his earlier account of how rights arise from desires (1983, pp. 109–112)).

2.4 Defining Personhood

Defenses of infanticide typically presuppose an understanding of personhood in which consciousness is necessary. Nicole Hassoun and Uriah Kriegel in their article "Consciousness and the Moral Permissibility of Infanticide" summarize their case against considering newborn babies as persons in the following way: "it is impermissible to intentionally kill a creature only if the creature is conscious; it is reasonable to believe that there is some time at which human infants are not conscious; therefore, it is reasonable to believe that it is permissible to intentionally kill some human infants" (2008, p. 45). The logic of their premises actually entails no limitation to only "some" infants. Similarly, according to Singer a being is a person if and only if the being has (1) an awareness of his or her own existence (2) over time and in different places with (3) the capacity to have wants and (4) plans for the future (Singer 1994, p. 218).

The necessity of self-awareness or consciousness for personhood is open to at least three interpretations. First, taken literally as stated—a being is a person if and only if it (actually) has awareness of his or her own existence, the definition would imply that we cease being persons each time we lose consciousness—with every surgery or every night sleep we lose rights. Taken literally the proposition that consciousness is necessary for personhood is ridiculous. This conception of personhood excludes not only the human newborn, but also mentally handicapped adults, if their disability is severe. No one believes it is permissible to kill human beings undergoing surgery or knocked out in a boxing match or rendered unconscious by a car accident, and yet in all these cases the human beings in question lack consciousness and self-awareness. One solution would be to say that such beings have *the potential* for self-awareness, but of course the same thing could be said of a human newborn, fetus, or embryo.

On a second view, *actual* self-awareness is not necessary for personhood, but rather the immediately exercisable *capacity* for self-awareness. A person fluent in German may be speaking English at the moment or may be asleep, but can switch in short order and actualize the dormant ability to speak German. The sleeping person can immediately exercise the capacity for consciousness simply by waking up, but the newborn cannot immediately exercise the capacity for self-awareness.

This understanding secures rights for normal sleeping adults but not for those in temporary comas, for they cannot *immediately actualize* their potential for self-awareness. Indeed, in some cases, it takes months or years before they again have the capacity for self-awareness, however, virtually no one holds that human beings in temporary comas do not deserve respect as persons.

On a third view, what is important is the possession of the "mental hardware" or current neural architecture (or something functionally equivalent) that enables self-awareness (Savulescu 2002). Even if you've never studied a word of German, and so cannot immediately actualize the potential you have to speak German, you have the capacity to learn the language if your brain functions in such a way that, given the right opportunity, you would learn German. The temporarily comatose human being retains capacity for self-awareness in the sense that this man or woman currently has the neural structure which is more than the mere *potential* for self-awareness possessed by the newborn or human fetus.

Capacity understood in this sense secures the right to life for some human beings in temporary comas, but not necessarily all. If someone's brain is badly injured in a car accident, in some cases the injured human being lacks functional neural hardware. Although it may not currently be possible given the state of our technology, let's say further that advanced medical techniques can repair the brain so that the injured person will again have the functional neural hardware. Prior to reparative surgery, the car accident victim is in the same position as the typical newborn in that he or she currently lacks functional neural capacity, but if all goes well, will later have the neural hardware. If such techniques were available, there would be no important difference between the personhood of the temporarily comatose of today and the car accident victim in the example. Thus, having the functional neural hardware needed for consciousness is not, in fact, essential for personhood.

Further, why should functional neural hardware be necessary for personhood? It is arbitrary simply to choose one necessary condition for self-awareness—neural structure—rather than others, such as being alive or having a rational nature. If any necessary condition for self-awareness is also sufficient, then again the living human infant possessing a rational nature should also be considered a person.

Another solution to the coma problem—which more broadly can be called the episodic problem—is to say that once a being becomes a person, that being does not lose this status until he or she no longer exists. Personhood, once attained with initial consciousness, cannot be lost until the end of the being's life.

However, in addition to being *ad hoc*, it is unclear why attaining consciousness should be decisive for personhood. Is personhood a reward for being conscious a short time? Why should a being who achieved consciousness but has permanently lost it be more valuable than a being who is about to achieve consciousness, which will be enjoyed over the course of a long life?

In any case, this response is not available to most advocates of this view, including Tooley and Singer, who hold that a human being *loses personhood* if consciousness is permanently lost, even if it was previously enjoyed. Say for example that both Clark and Greg are in comas. Although their comas are in all other respects identical, Clark needs Drug X to come out of his coma; Greg needs Drug Y. Luckily for Clark, someone invents Drug X and he is cured; but Drug Y has not yet been invented, so Greg's coma is considered permanent. In Singer and Tooley's view, Clark has a right to life because he is in a temporary coma but Greg does not have a right to life, *although both of them have been previously conscious*. So, in fact, it turns out that achieving consciousness is not morally decisive (nor is the dispositional desire to live which would be in *both* Greg and Clark while in their comas), but rather *the potentiality for future consciousness*. This leads to a contradiction. Defenders of infanticide deny the importance of potentiality in determining moral worth in the case of the human fetus or infant, but then must implicitly rely on the importance of potentiality in order to secure the right to life of those in temporary comas and in order to deny this right to those in permanent comas.

The second condition of Singer's definition of personhood—self-awareness over time and in different places—also raises difficulties. Imagine an alien perfectly suited to his or her present environment and therefore having no need, desire, or (given an advanced state of evolution in which unneeded abilities atrophy) capacity to move. Galen Strawson, in his book *Mental Reality*, imagines "weather watchers," stone-like creatures who have minds but exhibit no motion, nor any other behavior, whatsoever. They just sit on the coast and watch the weather. Why would such a being, perhaps much more rational than ourselves, not be a person? Strictly speaking, if self-awareness in different places is needed, the answer would be no. If a being is killed immediately *after* achieving self-awareness, is no person killed since self-awareness was not enjoyed over time? It seems odd that the necessary characteristic of personhood must be enjoyed over a particular amount of time in order to count.

The third condition—the capacity to have wants—also faces difficulties, depending on how "capacity" is defined. If capacity means a potentiality not realizable here and now but sometime in the future, then the human fetus would satisfy the definition. If capacity means a potentiality realizable immediately, then a human being in a temporary coma would not be a person. If capacity means currently having a functional brain that can give rise to desires, then those human beings whose brains are temporarily injured but who will recover do not count as persons.

Moreover, if unhappiness is not having your wants or desires fulfilled, then there is a powerful incentive either to satisfy your given desires or to minimize your desires as much as possible. Buddhism proposes this latter course of action. If Buddhists are right that the Buddha as well as other spiritual masters have reached a state of Nirvana—no longer desiring anything whatsoever and even extinguishing the capacity for desire—then either such mystics are no longer persons or having desires is not necessary for personhood. One could also imagine highly advanced aliens genetically engineered never to "want" precisely in order to realize the Buddhist dream. Or perhaps, if theists of a certain kind are right, then there are divine persons having all perfections, including the highest possible level of rationality, but entirely lacking the capacity to desire, since divine persons already enjoy and will always enjoy all perfections.

Singer can of course deny that there actually are Buddhist masters, perfectly satisfied aliens, or divine persons, but the point of the examples is conceptual. Such beings, if they were to exist, would obviously be persons, but would be excluded by definitions of personhood of defenders of infanticide, so such definitions are conceptually problematic. On the other hand, if we disallow such examples, then we should similarly disallow Tooley's talking kittens as well as numerous other analogies to be discussed later (e.g., space explorers and hooked up violinists) given on behalf of the pro-choice position.

If we drop the required "capacity" for desires in favor of *actually having* wants or desires, the same problems arise as with human beings sleeping, under the influence of drugs, or in temporary comas. None of these human beings, though clearly persons, has actual wants or desires.

In reply, one could argue that dispositional desires count for personhood rather than actual or potential desires. That is, when someone is sleeping, he or she retains dispositionally or habitually various desires and beliefs. Even while asleep, on drugs, or in a coma, a person desires and knows in this dispositional sense. We do not have to wake up each day and relearn how to read or rediscover our plans and desires. In sleep or in a coma, we have a dispositional desire to live that should be respected. But prior to conscious experience we do not.

A sophisticated version of this argument given by David Boonin in his book *A Defense of Abortion* will be dealt with more fully in chapter four, section 4.1.1, so here I will simply mention that Francis J. Beckwith has noted a difficulty with this view. Imagine two people in temporary comas, Bob and Stuart. Bob will come out of his coma but will have to relearn everything because of his severe brain trauma. He has no dispositional desires to live and therefore has no right to life.

> Stuart is in precisely the same position as Bob, except that Stuart will retain all his memories, prior abilities, etc. and it will take Stuart exactly the same amount of time to reacquire what he has lost as it will for Bob to acquire new memories and relearn old abilities and skills. If I understand Boonin's view of the right to life it would be permissible to kill Bob but not Stuart, even though the only difference between them would be that the latter will regain what he has lost while the former will gain memories he never had and many abilities he once mastered. Boonin clearly does not want to assert that it is prima facie permissible to kill a reversibly comatose person (123). Yet, given his position, it is prima facie permissible to kill a similarly situated reversibly comatose human being merely on the grounds that he will not be able to reacquire past traits and memories and he will have to relearn skills and abilities he possessed prior to his condition. It seems to me that the difference between Bob and Stuart carries no moral weight whatsoever.
>
> (Beckwith 2006, p. 184)

The prospect of "relearning everything" is daunting in the case of adults (but so would be the rehab to reacquire everything that was learned) so our intuitions may not be as clear as Beckwith would like. However, if we were to change the example slightly and make Bob and Stuart young children, the point may be even easier to see. Particularly in the case of young children, where the skills and memories lost would be very minimal (since the skills and memories were relatively undeveloped to begin with), it is clear that the distinction between a human being in a temporary coma who will recover old desires and a human being in a temporary coma who will acquire new desires is of no real importance. Just because the 1-year-old Stuart will eventually be able to recall a few memories from the crib, and 1-year-old Bob will not, hardly justifies the difference between having and not having the right to life.

The fourth condition—planning for the future—also faces difficulties. One can easily imagine beings so powerfully rational that they do not "plan" and have no need for a capacity (in any sense) to plan. To plan, by definition, involves discursive reasoning, the considering of premises, and the working out of likely conclusions, rather than understanding intuitively and immediately, and, therefore, without planning, all that is entailed by any "direction of travel." The difference between human reasoning and the reasoning of these beings could be compared to the difference between a child learning to read and a sophisticated adult reader. Children learning to read must sound out each letter, piece together syllables, and then finally, slowly pronounce the entire word. Often, this laborious process is so slow, and takes so much effort, that beginner readers forget the words at the start of a sentence by the time they reach the end of the sentence. In contrast, an advanced reader can read and understand not only entire words at a glance but many phrases and even short sentences. They read. They don't sound out. The difference between the discursive human reasoning and the intuitive reasoning of the beings we are imagining here would be even more pronounced. Even though such beings having intuitive reasoning can act, they do not *plan for the future*, since this implies gathering bits of information, trying to understand how various bits of information relate to one another, and then finally formulating a plan for the future based on the information gathered, collated, and weighed in a prudential judgment. Rather, such beings immediately see and understand the implications not only of reality, but also of what reality would be if they choose one course of action or another. Such beings would not plan, but they are clearly persons, and if they are clearly persons, then Singer's definition of person is incorrect.

Ironically, Singer's definition of personhood fails in part because it is deeply anthropocentric. His "speciesist" account of personhood assumes that the norms of psychology, practical reasoning, and time–space experience typical of healthy, adult human beings must apply to all persons. John Locke was writing about personhood as an account of human *responsibility* not of personal *moral worth*. As Patrick Kain points out with respect to Immanuel Kant, and the same holds true for Locke, "personhood and responsibility does not entail that each person acts or has acted, or that each is always able to act; it only entails that *when* or *if* a person does act, she may be held responsible for her actions" (2009, p. 66).

2.5 Seriously Ill Newborns

Some people oppose killing healthy newborns, but make an exception for killing disabled babies. In their *Hasting's Center Report* article "Ending the Life of a Newborn: The Groningen Protocol," Hilde Lindemann and Marian Verkerk support those who "responsibly end the lives of severely impaired newborns" of various kinds suffering from serious illness (2008, p. 42). Their argument is fairly straightforward and similar in form to the argument in favor of euthanasia generally (another practice legally accepted in the Netherlands). They note that most people already sanction removal of life support from severely handicapped babies who have no chance of survival (Group 1):

> Group 2 consists of infants who "may survive after a period of intensive treatment, but expectations regarding their future condition are very grim." They include infants with severe brain abnormalities or extensive organ damage caused by lack of oxygen. The dilemma here is whether these infants are so badly off that they should be allowed to die.
>
> (Lindemann & Verkerk 2008, p. 42)

In the United States and Europe, there is a consensus that it is permissible to withdraw or withhold treatment from such children, allowing them to die. "In the Netherlands, however, if neither withholding nor withdrawing intensive treatment will result in a speedy death, the unbearable suffering of the infant is seen as a compelling reason for the doctor to end its life directly" (Lindemann & Verkerk 2008, p. 42). Group 3 are seriously disabled infants who could survive into adulthood with conditions causing terrible suffering (Lindemann & Verkerk 2008, p. 44). The Groningen Protocol applies to babies in all three groups, allowing for intentional killing of newborns, contingent upon both parents giving informed consent, a certain diagnosis of "hopeless and unbearable suffering" being confirmed by at least one independent doctor, and also the consent of the physician who will kill the baby. From Lindemann and Verkerk's perspective, babies in Group 3 have the most pressing need to be killed, since they could survive into adulthood with their terrible conditions (2008, p. 46).

Lindemann and Verkerk defend the Groningen Protocol for killing newborns, which they argue has been misunderstood by errors in linguistic translation as well as in cultural misunderstandings of the Dutch context. At times, their defense of infanticide seems to rest on a moral relativism wherein infanticide is permissible in Holland, but perhaps not elsewhere. Moral relativism is typically not presupposed in discussions of infanticide, since relativism opens the door to approval of sex-selection abortion and infanticide of baby girls, as practiced in some parts of the world for cultural reasons.

Even aside from presupposing relativism, the other problems with Lindemann and Verkerk's defense are foundational, rather than a matter of clarifying, for instance, that not only babies with spina bifida, but also many other babies will be subject to the protocol. For example, Lindemann and Verkerk presuppose the permissibility of physician-assisted suicide and voluntary euthanasia, and they do not answer the important objections raised against such practices (see, for example, Keown 2002). They take for granted that severe suffering (understood as physical pain and/or psychological agony) renders the life of the one who suffers worthless by presupposing body–self dualism. However, there is good reason to question dualistic conceptions of the personal "self" set against the person's embodied existence (see, for example, Lee & George 2007). If all human persons have intrinsic value, and if a person's *life* is simply nothing other than the *person* in his or her bodily dimension, then all human lives, even those who severely suffer, have intrinsic value. To cite one more problematic assumption of this defense of killing disabled newborns, the authors repeatedly offer a false alternative: either allow the baby to suffer or intentionally kill the infant. No mention is made of a third alternative: making use of drugs to relieve suffering, even if the dosage must be high enough to induce deep sleep.

Lindemann and Verkerk recognize a significant objection to their defense of infanticide that some babies, if allowed to live, would be like most other adults glad they were not killed at birth.

> It is of course true that some of these babies—those, for example, who face complete lifelong dependency—might, if kept alive, judge as adults that their lives had been worth something to them. Much would depend, one supposes, on how much pain and other kinds of suffering they had to endure to get to adulthood. But that consideration is no reason to proscribe all life-ending interventions on the basis of future suffering.
>
> (2008, p. 48)

Why not? Empirical evidence shows that the overwhelming majority of adults suffering from serious illness do not kill themselves. These people have presumably known good health at some point in their lives, and so they suffer additionally (as children from Group 3 would not) in missing what they have lost. We have good reason to suppose that children from Group 3 would, as adults, value their lives, a consideration that should not be simply dismissed. Justifying infanticide in such cases amounts to killing a person against their (presumed) consent.

Lindemann and Verkerk also falsely assume that the withdrawal or withholding of life support for an uncomprehending patient of any age depends upon a judgment that the patient's life is no longer of value. However, the decision not to administer or to remove life-sustaining treatment does not need to rest on the assumption that the person's life or the person himself or herself is not valuable. If the burdens of a treatment outweigh its benefits, in the view of whoever has authority for the patient's care, then the treatment need not be administered or may be withdrawn without any recourse to beliefs that they or their lives are worthless. Of course, the patient's condition will partially determine the degree to which any given treatment is beneficial and burdensome (Keown 2002). However, the appropriate question is whether a given *treatment* is more beneficial than burdensome, not whether a person's *life* is beneficial or burdensome (*Lebensunwertes Leben*).

2.6 Arbitrary Limits?

Defenses of infanticide typically assume that in most cases in which infanticide is desirable it will be apparent shortly after birth (Tooley 1972, p. 64; see also Singer 2000, p. 162). However, in many cases, the extent of medical disabilities of handicapped children is not realized in a short time after birth. A severely disabled child and a normal newborn may not display notable differences at birth or in the first few months of life outside the womb. Only as the months and even years go on, as the handicapped child does not show signs of developing even slowly, can the extent of neurological damage be determined. So the capricious limit of one week, proposed by Tooley, or one month, proposed by Singer, would not even accomplish the goal of sparing the parents of disabled offspring the difficulties of raising a disabled child. Sometimes parents only discover the depth of such illnesses later, when it would be "too late" according to Tooley's or Singer's standards, to terminate the child.

Bolder proposals have been brought forward to extend the permissible time period for killing of human beings after birth. Although some claim evidence of self-awareness only 12–14 days after birth, Hassoun and Kriegel also offer what they take to be another plausible cut off point for infanticide:

> [I]t is quite plausible to take mirror self-recognition to be *evidence for* the presence of self-awareness. The question we want to ask ourselves is at what age humans develop the ability for mirror self-recognition. The evidence suggests that humans develop the capacity for mirror self-recognition between the ages of eighteen months and twenty-four months.
>
> (2008, p. 49)

Although almost everyone rejects the killing of innocent children up to two years of age, the view that personhood requires conscious self-awareness pushes us to this absurd conclusion, which is good reason to reject this view of personhood.

The conception of personhood used by defenders of infanticide also leads them to posit arbitrary deadlines to separate who may live from who may be killed. Indeed setting the age for voting or driving at 18 or 16 is indeed arbitrary, for many people are ready for these activities earlier and some not until later. However, in matters of life and death we must do better than picking a random cut off point. Life itself is at stake, the existence of innocent human beings, and so a vision of personhood that rests on the arbitrary decisions of the powerful against the weak cannot be in conformity with the demands of justice or equality.

Indeed, taken to their logical conclusion, the views advocated by defenders of infanticide are so radical that they lead to implications that virtually no one can accept. In his book, *The Ethics of Killing: Problems at the Margins of Life*, Jeff McMahan comes to the conclusion that it is morally permissible to kill a healthy orphaned infant in order to use his or her organs to attempt to save the lives of other human beings (2002, pp. 359, 360). He calls the scenario, "Healthy Newborn."

> A woman dies in childbirth leaving a very premature but healthy infant, just a few hours old. The child's biological father died months ago and neither he nor the mother had any living relatives. Both were reclusive and had no friends; hence there is no one who is specially related, even indirectly, to the infant. Suppose there are four children in the same hospital, all of whom are three years old and need an organ transplant within the next twenty-four hours in order to survive. Because these children's organs have been impaired by illness, it is not possible to wait for one to die and use his or her organs to save the others; nor is it possible to sacrifice one (say, by lottery) to save the other three. But the newborn infant has the right tissue type and its organs could be used to save all four.
>
> (2007, p. 22)

The conclusion that healthy newborns may be killed to harvest their organs causes McMahan "significant misgivings and considerable unease," but he is not troubled enough to abandon his theory of moral status. If his conclusions were correct, it would seem to follow that it is *morally required*, and not merely permissible, if other things are equal, to kill the healthy, orphaned newborn if its organs could help save a single person. It is not as if *four* children must be helped by the sacrifice, and helping just two or one would be insufficient. And no reason is given to think that only saving a person's life could justify killing the healthy newborn. Hopes of medical breakthroughs to cure non-lethal diseases would be sufficient reason for vivisection of infants. Why shouldn't helping a "real" person in any way be a sufficient justification for killing the healthy, orphaned newborn non-person? Indeed, if a newborn immediately after birth is less a person than a calf, pig, or chicken (Singer

1993, p. 151), then infanticide should be no more difficult to justify than painlessly killing an animal for food.

These dubious conclusions apply not merely to the human infant, but also to adult humans who, because they are mentally handicapped, function at the same level as infants. Indeed, killing handicapped human beings becomes governed by the norms equally applicable to painlessly killing animals (McMahan 2003, p. 531). Unless "real" human persons, for instance relatives or benefactors, object—a caveat equally applicable to painlessly killing animals—one could, indeed should, kill mentally handicapped women and men for their organs or simply to alleviate burdens on others. There are approximately 100,000 people on organ transplant waiting lists in the United States alone, but only 10,000 to 20,000 organ donations per year (Harter 2008, p. 155). On the supposition that personhood requires a level of rational functioning beyond what a healthy newborn enjoys, the severely mentally handicapped provide an untapped resource for curing the ailments of those who are deemed "real" human persons.

Needless to say, questions and critical responses have bedeviled defenses of infanticide. Most people who defend the moral permissibility of abortion do not also defend infanticide. Many of these people hold that abortion is permissible from conception until birth but not afterwards. Newborn infants, on this view, should not be intentionally killed even if unwanted by their parents, even if born into tragic situations, even if conceived by rape or incest, even if their prospects in life look dim. However, a human being in utero, in the very same or even in less dire circumstances, may be aborted. In the next chapter, we will be looking at arguments in favor of this view that human beings outside the womb should not be killed; however, human beings in utero may be aborted at any stage of pregnancy.

3 Does Personhood Begin at Birth?

Planned Parenthood and the National Abortion and Reproductive Rights Action League (NARAL), as well as many pro-choice politicians, hold that abortion ought to be legally permissible through all nine months of pregnancy, but that infanticide should be illegal. Many defenders of abortion hold a parallel ethical position, that abortion is also morally permissible throughout all stages of pregnancy, but that infanticide is ethically wrong. This perspective corrects the pro-life view (to be presented in chapter five) by providing criteria for distinguishing persons from mere humans, and yet also disagrees with an expansion of "reproductive rights" to include infanticide. This chapter presents arguments in favor of this view and offers possible responses both from the perspective of an advocate of infanticide and from the perspective of a defender of prenatal human life.

In her influential articles "The Personhood Argument in Favor of Abortion" and "On the Moral and Legal Status of Abortion," Mary Anne Warren draws a distinction between a "human being" and a "person." Human beings, those beings genetically classified in the species *Homo sapiens*, may or may not be persons. Persons, including human beings in the "moral" sense, are bearers of rights and always merit our consideration and respect. Mere human beings are not members of the moral community simply by virtue of their humanity. Persons, however, have rights that must be respected, including the right to life.

3.1 Distinguishing Humans from Persons

What distinguishes mere human beings or "potential" persons from "actual" or "real" persons? Warren offers five different criteria by which we might separate these two classes of beings (1973, p. 263). It is not necessary to have all these traits to be a person, but any being lacking all these traits is certainly not a person. First, persons have, "consciousness of objects and events external and/or internal to themselves, in particular the capacity to feel pain" (Warren 1973, p. 263). Human beings who lack this capacity for consciousness, particularly those who lack the capacity to experience pain, are not persons. Second, persons can reason. They have the "developed capacity to solve new and relatively complex problems" (Warren 1973, p. 263). Potential persons, on the other hand, cannot function in this way. Third, persons have self-motivated activity, that is, "activity which is relatively independent of either genetic or direct external control" (Warren 1973, p. 263). Potential persons cannot control themselves to the requisite degree. Fourth, persons possess "the capacity to communicate, by whatever means, messages of an indefinite variety of types, that is, not just with an indefinite number of possible contents, but on indefinitely many topics" (Warren 1973, p. 263). Potential persons can only communicate very little, or sometimes not at all. Finally, persons have, "the presence of self-concepts, and self-awareness, either individual or racial, or both" (Warren 1973, p. 263). Mere human beings lack these self-concepts. This last criterion of personhood does not differ significantly from what Tooley offered in the previous chapter, but the other criteria are new.

For Warren, the first and second conditions, namely sensitivity to pain and reasoning ability, may be sufficient for personhood, but if a being were to lack all five characteristics that being would certainly not be a person (Warren 1973, p. 263), though the being might be a potential person. Here the distinction between mere human beings and persons is more stringent than Tooley's, since Warren adds several characteristics that are necessary for personhood in addition to consciousness. For Warren, severely handicapped human beings, humans injured in the process of birth or even by an accident later in life, are not persons if they have permanently lost consciousness (Warren 1973, pp. 263–264). Hence, Warren's criteria would exclude not just all human beings prior to birth but also some human beings long after birth.

Should a conflict arise between the rights of persons to health, happiness, or freedom and the rights of potential persons, the rights of persons prevail. The right of a woman to an abortion always outweighs whatever right to live ascribed to a human fetus, even a fully developed one (Warren 1973, p. 264).

It might be objected that even if the human fetus is not a person, it is at least a *potential* person and the rights of a potential person should count for something. It may even be the case, in certain circumstances, that the rights of a potential person outweigh the rights of a person. Warren rejects such considerations by means of analogy:

> Suppose that [a] space explorer falls into the hands of an alien culture, whose scientists decide to create a few hundred thousand or more human beings, by breaking his body into its component cells, and using these to create fully developed human beings, with, of course, his genetic code. We may imagine that each of these newly created men will have all of the original man's abilities, skills, knowledge,

and so on, and also have an individual self-concept; in short, that each of them will be a *bona fide* (though hardly unique) person. Imagine that the whole project will take only seconds, and that its chances of success are extremely high, and that our explorer knows all of this, and also knows that these people will be treated fairly. I maintain that in such a situation he would have every right to escape if he could, and thus to deprive all of these potential people of their potential lives; for his right to life outweighs all of theirs together, in spite of the fact that they are all genetically human, all innocent, and all have a very high probability of becoming people very soon, if only he refrains from acting.

(1973, pp. 265–266)

With the advent of human cloning, Warren's analogy is not as outlandish as it might seem at first consideration. Each cell of every human body can be cloned to make a new human being, an identical twin who differs in age and life experience, but who shares DNA with its original human "parent." May we violate the rights of one actual person, the space explorer, in order to secure the right to life of the potential persons virtually present in each cell of the space explorer's body? If our answer is no, then the rights of potential persons, even thousands of innocent potential persons, do not outweigh the rights of a single actual person.

3.2 Abortion Yes, Infanticide No

As Warren realizes, the conception of personhood advocated here would also exclude newborn babies, and so on the basis of this reasoning it should be concluded that killing a newborn infant is not murder, since infanticide is not killing a person, but only a human being (1973, p. 266). Nevertheless, Warren differs from advocates of infanticide in coming to the conclusion that although newborns are not persons strictly speaking, infanticide is nevertheless wrong. Why? Infanticide is wrong according to Warren first of all because even if biological parents don't want the child, other people do (Warren 1973, p. 266). In 2002, for example, there were more than 1.5 million couples waiting to adopt children in the United States alone. Given the increasing fertility problems of Western societies, due to a variety of cultural and possibly environmental causes, infants of all races are in great demand. Now since it is generally wrong to destroy something that another person greatly wants, even if you don't happen to greatly want it, it is wrong to destroy a newborn who is wanted by others.

Second, Warren notes that most people don't want infants destroyed (Warren 1973, p. 266). If people want to protect newborn babies, and are willing to pay for orphanages or other needed care, then infants ought not be destroyed but rather protected. Thus, not just various individuals, but society as a whole desires for newborns not to be destroyed but protected by law and welcomed into life. However, Warren holds that killing unwanted or defective infants born into a society that doesn't value newborns would be permissible. The rationale appears to be that in such a society others would not want the newborns (Warren 1973, p. 267). However, our society does value newborns and so killing newborns in our context would be impermissible.

For Warren, however, the key difference between abortion and infanticide is that the human fetus resides within the woman and so violates her rights to freedom, happiness, and self-determination. If, somehow, removal of the human being in utero could take place without killing, killing would not be permissible, just as it is not permissible after birth (Warren 1973, p. 267).

Taking a similar position, and offering further reasons to distinguish between killing infants and killing human fetuses, H. Tristram Engelhardt in his article, "Sanctity of Life and the Concept of a Person," follows Warren in marking the distinction between persons and mere human beings in such a way that renders newborn human beings non-persons. Engelhardt speaks of a "social concept of person." He invokes this social concept of a person in some instances where a human being is not strictly speaking a person but should be accorded the social status of personhood anyway. Why grant such status to newborns? Engelhardt offers several reasons (Engelhardt 2000, p. 81): First, the infant is biologically human and so deserves a modicum of respect. Second, newborns are also able to engage in a minimum of social interaction. Third, a human fetus can survive regardless of social recognition; a newborn cannot survive regardless of social recognition. Fourth, forbidding infanticide helps preserve trust in families, nurtures important virtues of care and solicitude towards the weak, and assures the healthy development of children. Fifth, Engelhardt notes that there is value in protecting whatever looks and acts in human fashion (2000, p. 82). Finally, human infants will become persons strictly speaking and actions taken against infants injure the persons they will become (Engelhardt 2000, p. 82).

Why not include human beings in utero as persons in this social sense? Engelhardt provides several answers. Abortion aids the convenience of women and families, prevents the birth of infants with serious genetic diseases, helps control population growth, secures a woman's right to choose freely concerning her body, as well as secures a woman's freedom to determine whether she will become a mother. Thus, for both Warren and Engelhardt, although neither a human fetus nor a newborn are strictly speaking persons, newborns should not be killed, but abortion is permissible.

3.3 Critiquing the Conventional View

Various efforts to approve abortion but condemn infanticide often suffer from a two-fold difficulty. Arguments against infanticide often apply equally well to abortion while arguments in favor of abortion often apply equally well to infanticide. Thus, both those who are pro-life as well as advocates of infanticide agree that the conventional view is incoherent. For instance, infanticide is wrong in Warren's view because even if biological parents don't want the child, other people do. Since 1.5 million couples are waiting to adopt children in the United States alone, infanticide is impermissible. A difficulty for those holding the conventional pro-choice view is that this very same reasoning would render not only infanticide but also abortion impermissible. Not only would infanticide prevent these 1.5 million couples from being able to adopt those children killed, but also abortion prevents the adoption of all those who are aborted. Thus, Warren has provided us with reason to reject both abortion and infanticide. Warren's other argument against infanticide, that most people don't want infants harmed or destroyed, could also apply to abortion. Most people support the idea of providing good prenatal care for pregnant women, most people believe it is particularly bad to harm a pregnant woman, and the vast majority of people feel very uncomfortable with abortion even if they believe abortion should be legal. Many people oppose all abortions, and among those who do not, many of these want abortion to be safe, legal, and *rare*. Very few indeed see abortion as anything more than a tragic last resort, let alone a positive good. The reason for such judgments, as well as the instinctive emotional reaction of most people to seeing pictures of aborted fetuses, is that the human being in utero, even if not accorded full personhood, nevertheless is in some important sense valuable, important, and seen as a good by society. Obviously, not every single person in society shares this general concern, but the same may also be said about concern for newborns.

The alleged differences between abortion and infanticide supplied by Engelhardt are invoked to answer the question: Why not also grant the fetus this social conception of personhood, if the newborn has this status? However, his reasons for opposing infanticide also apply to abortion. After all, if an infant deserves some modicum of respect because it is genetically human, why shouldn't a human fetus conceived by human parents and within a human mother, belonging to the species *Homo sapiens* just as much as any newborn, also merits respect? Although a newborn is able to engage in a minimum of social interaction, these interactions do not differ in any significant respect from the social interaction of a fetus at a late stage of development. What is the crucial difference in social interaction between an 8-month-old human fetus and a newborn? Both can react to a stimulus provided by light or touch; both can invoke warm feelings in adults (witness sonograms on refrigerators); both can cry, suck thumbs, and open eyes. Although Engelhard notes that a human fetus can survive regardless of social recognition and that a baby cannot survive regardless of social recognition, one wonders why social recognition should play such a significant role. After all, one sign of a corrupt society (e.g., anti-Semitism) is that such societies do not grant social recognition to all. In any case, our society does grant some social recognition to prenatal human beings in a number of ways through the law (e.g., California provides free prenatal care, public signs in bars warn of the effects of alcohol on the preborn) and through acknowledging miscarriage, especially late-term miscarriage, as a grave loss. The murder of Laci Peterson and her unborn son Connor resulted in a charge of double murder. It is especially strange that the relative independence of the human fetus (who doesn't need societal recognition to survive) is now used as an argument *against* granting preborn human beings a right to life, while most arguments for abortion, for example from viability, claim that the dependence of the fetus undermines the human being in utero's right to life.

For those who want to defend abortion but condemn infanticide, Engelhardt's arguments provide little support because his reasons for opposing infanticide apply equally well to abortion. Although it is claimed that forbidding infanticide preserves trust in families, one could also argue that some children would be "freaked out" to learn of a brother or sister aborted by their mother. Although Engelhardt points out that forbidding infanticide nurtures important virtues of care and solicitude towards the weak, one could argue that preserving unborn human life also nurtures these virtues towards those who are even weaker. If banning infanticide contributes to ensure the healthy development of children, why wouldn't the same be true of banning abortion?

Engelhardt holds that there is value in protecting whatever looks and acts in a human fashion, and thus infanticide should be forbidden. Again it is unclear why this same point might not also be made in respect to abortion. As abortion defender Judith Jarvis Thomson points out:

> I am inclined to think also that we shall probably have to agree that the fetus has already become a human person well before birth. Indeed it comes as a surprise when one first learns how early in its life it begins to acquire human characteristics. By the tenth week, for example, it already has a face, arms and legs, fingers and toes; it has internal organs and brain activity is detectable.
>
> (1971, pp. 47–48)

As ultrasound technology makes clear, the human fetus from a fairly early stage is easily recognizable as a human being.

Engelhardt's final plea for not putting unwanted infants to death is that with luck they will become persons in the full sense and that if we harm them now we will also injure the persons they will become later, but these rationales apply also to unborn human beings. If not killed in utero, the vast majority of human fetuses will become human adults and, similar to infants, injuries sustained to these human beings at the beginning of life will sometimes remain injuries on through adulthood. Fetal alcohol syndrome and 'crack babies' have taught us this tragic lesson in all too vivid detail. In sum, Engelhardt's rationale for condemning infanticide provides reasons to question the legitimacy of abortion.

On the other hand, defenders of putting newborns to death will find in Engelhardt's justification of abortion an even greater justification for infanticide. If abortion secures the convenience of women and families, the same thing could be said of infanticide, since for most women (and even more clearly for their families) a child is much more inconvenient *after birth* due to multiple nighttime feedings, frequent cries, and dirty diapers. Before birth, none of these inconveniences are in play. Of course, adoption can also eliminate these inconveniences, but if the newborn is not a being worthy of respect, there is no reason to think one has an obligation to dispose of a newborn in one way rather than another. Further, adoption could be considered burdensome to birth mothers in a way that infanticide is not, for with adoption a grown child may seek to establish unwanted contact with his or her mother (though contemporary adoptions practices can block this possibility). Abortion can indeed end the existence of human fetuses with serious genetic diseases; but infanticide can eliminate not only newborns with genetic defects (pathologies whose existence and severity is often more easily ascertained *after* birth) but also the significant number of infants who become injured and handicapped, often seriously, in the process of birth itself by, for example, oxygen deprivation.

Abortion secures a woman's freedom to determine whether she will become a mother, but so also would infanticide (as well as adoption). Following birth, with greater knowledge about her offspring and a more realistic sense of how this newborn impacts her life, a woman would be better able to make a truly informed choice about whether she wanted to take on the burdens of motherhood.

Abortion can help control population, but infanticide accomplishes the same goal more effectively. Though exact numbers remain a matter of controversy, a significant percentage of all newly conceived human beings spontaneously miscarry anyway, so abortion in such cases is unnecessary. If population reduction is the goal, infanticide achieves this goal more effectively than abortion. Biologically considered, there is an asymmetry between the reproductive potentiality of women and men. A man can father hundreds or even thousands of children, but a woman can give birth to only a small fraction as many. Imagine two boats stranded on separate islands. On the first island are stranded a men's soccer team and one female coach; on the second island, a women's soccer team and one male coach. If the inhabitants of both islands seek to reproduce maximally, it is clear which island will have the greater population. Therefore, reducing the number of females is a more effective means of reducing population than simply reducing the number of males and females equally. Since a child's gender is more easily determined following birth than prior to birth, especially in low-income countries without widespread access to ultrasound, infanticide targeting female babies would be a more effective way to reduce population than abortion of equal numbers of males and females.

So if neither human fetuses nor newborns count as persons in a strict sense, and all the reasons given by Engelhardt for not counting human beings in utero as social persons apply also to newborns, we are left with a question. Why should human infants count as persons, even in a social sense?

The one true difference that Engelhardt (as well as Warren) appeal to that actually does distinguish infanticide from abortion is that with infanticide the human being is no longer in the women's body and with abortion the young human being is still within the woman's body.

However, if a human newborn is not a person, indeed if Warren is right that a newborn is no more person-like than "a newborn guppy" or "the average fish" (1973, pp. 264–265), then a condemnation of infanticide is difficult to sustain. After all, a fish's location is irrelevant to its non-existent right to life. If the third trimester human fetus or newborn is less of a person than the average fish, then surely there is reason to allow infanticide in light of the demands infants make. If a fish were to wake you up several times a night, demanding food or a change of water, and on the horizon you knew you had to pay thousands of dollars each year, for 18 years, to keep the fish alive, would anyone blame you for killing it? So what if your neighbors or hundreds of others want your fish? Who could seriously disagree with the proposal that your fish is your fish to raise and to love, or to kill and to eat, as you see fit?

However, one might respond that according to Warren, the important difference between a newborn and the human fetus is that the former is not within her body and the latter is within her body. So, in the case of abortion, but not infanticide, her bodily rights are in play. It is these bodily rights that make abortion permissible but not infanticide; for in the case of infanticide the bodily rights are no longer at issue. In other words, on this view the personhood of the fetus is not denied. Rather, the right to detach oneself from the fetus is asserted. This powerful defense of the conventional view—from a woman's rights regarding her body—will be examined later in detail in chapter six.

However, this response is unavailable to Warren. A woman's right to abortion, according to Warren, does not rest on her bodily rights alone but also on other considerations, such as happiness and freedom that extends beyond simply concern for physical well-being (1996, p. 88).

Since the rights of actual persons (not *just* bodily rights) always infinitely outweigh the rights of potential persons, the fact that the bodily rights of the woman are no longer in play in the case of infanticide does not undermine her right to choose to kill the newborn who is, on her account, merely a potential person with the moral status of a guppy.

In later work, responding to the criticism that she must, to be consistent, either abandon a permissive position on abortion or embrace infanticide (Card 2000), Warren adds two other reasons to distinguish abortion from infanticide. The first is that humans that are not yet persons become persons through a long period of dependence and interaction with moral agents who are persons in the full sense. If we want there to be moral agents in the future, if we want infants and children to have any chance at good lives, we must value the lives and well-being of infants and young children, even though strictly speaking they are not persons (Warren 1997, pp. 164–165).

This reasoning does not exclude the selective choice of infanticide or child killing before speech emerges. Of course, if we collectively want human moral agents to exist in the future, then we cannot kill *all* newborns or older children just as we cannot abort every human fetus. However, like abortion as now practiced, the killing of millions of infants and children who cannot yet speak is perfectly compatible with the general continuation of the human race and desiring that those selected to continue have good lives.

Warren's second reason for distinguishing abortion and infanticide rests on the mental differences between a newborn and a human fetus as established by behavioral and neuro-physiological evidence (Warren 2000, p. 355). The argument seems to be that although at the end of pregnancy there is no significant difference between a human being in utero and a newly born human being, earlier in pregnancy, at the stage where sentience is just emerging, the differences between a newborn and human fetus are significant. So, there is an important difference between abortion and infanticide.

Although there clearly is a difference between fetal sentience early in pregnancy and the sentience of a newborn human being, this difference does not help to mark a difference between abortion and infanticide. As Warren tacitly admits, there is no significant difference in sentience between a human fetus a day before birth and the same human being 24 hours later following birth. In order to show a difference between abortion and infanticide, the defender of abortion must show that there is an important difference between abortion and infanticide *in this case*, and not merely recast the objection into one more easily handled, that is, one involving the difference between abortion of an incipiently sentient human fetus (perhaps as early as eight weeks) and infanticide. There are clearly differences in development between *these* cases, but pointing this out does not answer the question about what is the difference between abortion at 30 weeks into pregnancy and infanticide of an infant prematurely born at the same time.

In addition, although the behavioral and neuropsychological evidence does suggest that age and physical development of a human being are linked with sentience and other mental development, this link undermines any necessary difference in sentience between a human being pre-birth and post-birth. Consider for example, an infant born prematurely at 30 weeks gestation and a human fetus at 40 weeks gestation just prior to full-term birth. All the evidence would suggest that the human fetus in this situation is *more developed* in terms of sentience and mental ability than the newborn. If the reasons adduced by Warren were true, abortion would be more difficult to justify than infanticide in such cases. Given that more than 10% of births in the United States are premature, such situations where a given human infant is less developed than a given human fetus are quite common. Yet it can also happen that in the same hospital, on one floor medical personnel work frantically to save the life of a premature newborn, while on another floor an abortionist aborts a more fully developed human being in utero. Since sentience and mental development do not mark any necessary difference between pre-birth and post-birth human beings, the only difference remaining is location.

A final reason given by Warren to distinguish infanticide from abortion is on the basis of the development of moral agency (1997, pp. 164–165). Human beings only become moral agents through a long period of development and dependence upon other moral agents.

> For this reason, it is both impractical and emotionally abhorrent to deny full moral status to sentient human beings who have not yet achieved (or who have irreparably lost) the capacity for moral agency. If we want there to be human beings in the world in the future, and if we want them to have any chance to lead good lives, then we must at least value the lives and well-being of infants and young children. Fortunately, instinct, reason, and culture jointly ensure that most of us regard infants and young children as human beings to whom we can have obligations as binding as those we have to human beings who are moral agents.
>
> (Warren 1997, pp. 164–165)

These considerations do not provide a good rationale for according a right to live to human infants. Not everyone finds infanticide abhorrent, so those that do find the killing of infants abhorrent could simply refrain from the practice. If we want there to be human beings in the world in the future, then we do not need to value the lives and well-being of all infants and all young children, but rather only some—for example, those infants and young children who are wanted by moral agents.

Even if Warren's considerations did work, they could indicate that human beings prior to birth should also be accorded the rights of moral agents. Many people find denying rights to children abhorrent, but many people also find abortion abhorrent. It is true that "most of us" regard infants and young children as human beings to whom we can have obligations, but in certain times and places "most of us" would have said the same thing about human beings prior to birth. In any case, a majority of people can be wrong.

3.4 Is Personhood a Matter of Location?

Warren's defense of abortion and rejection of infanticide rests on making birth the practical, though not the theoretical, way of distinguishing mere humans from persons. In other words, although *theoretically* newborn babies are not persons any more than are human beings in utero (or a guppy), nevertheless *practically* speaking a human being is granted the rights of a person at birth and so can no longer be killed. Birth is the moment when a human being begins to have rights, including the right to life that must be respected. (Of course, for Warren and Engelhardt, a newborn baby is not really a person but nevertheless should be treated as if he or she were a person because of prudential considerations.) Unlike the having of a "concept of self," birth is an empirically verifiable event. Unlike the "ability to reason" criterion, the birth criterion would not keep severely mentally handicapped persons and the senile elderly from having a right to life. Unlike self-awareness, birth is a definitive event that one can easily recognize. And at birth potential conflicts between the bodily rights of the mother and the human fetus end (Green 2002).

However, one is or is not a person regardless of location within or not within another person's body. Why should the personhood of a human being be diminished or even extinguished because he or she is within another person's body? Imagine the consequences of such a view for dentists, surgeons, and men engaged in sexual intercourse. It seems strange that being just inside or outside the cervix makes a difference to whether one counts as a person.

Marking personhood by existence outside the mother (be it through birth, cesarean section, or artificial womb) also commits one to a conception of personhood plagued by what might be called the "episodic problem." Whatever personhood is, it surely cannot be something that comes and goes episodically. We do not cease to be persons when we are sleeping or in surgery even though Green recognizes that we do not in such times have a concept of ourselves. Why? Because it would be absurd to have this most important of properties—the right to life that comes with personhood—come and go and then come back again episodically. However, if one attempts to make birth the moment when personhood arrives because at birth the young human being exists outside the mother, one runs into this episodic problem. A newly conceived human being would be a person if conceived outside the womb (ironically with a much smaller chance of reaching adulthood than a human being conceived normally, who wouldn't on this view count as a person) but when put into the womb this human embryo would temporarily lose personhood only to regain it again later after leaving the womb. During open fetal surgery, the human fetus is sometimes brought outside the uterus. Determining personhood by existence outside the womb commits one to the implausible view that in such cases the human fetus is a non-person who becomes a person while outside his or her mother's body, and then becomes a non-person again when returned to the uterus only to become a person once again at birth. Repeated surgeries would multiply the confused personhood of the fetal patient.

Richard Doerflinger also notes that birth is not so definitive and easily recognized as it may seem since the birthing process can extend over hours, and even days (Doerflinger 2002, p. 31). Before making birth the all-important cut off point for personhood, an important question needs to be adequately answered: Is there really any important difference in the personhood of a human being one minute before birth and one minute after? Why should a tiny human embryo conceived in a Petri dish have personhood simply because it is not in the uterus, while a fully viable human fetus just before birth does not?

As Doerflinger suggests, birth itself is a process of exiting the mother, and one must wonder at what point in this process personhood appears. Is leaving the uterus the important moment or leaving the vaginal canal? Must the offspring be entirely outside the womb or would the exiting of the head alone grant personhood? What if the entire baby was born but the doctor held a single foot within the mother? What if the entire body of the baby is outside the mother via breach birth but the head alone remains inside? Today, these questions are anything but merely theoretical because of the ongoing political, legal, and moral disputes about partial-birth abortion. But even some of those who approve of partial-birth abortion have noted that location makes no relevant difference for personhood. Lawrence H. Tribe, in reference to a proposed law banning partial-birth abortion in some circumstances, writes:

> The proposed statute therefore seeks to make the legality of the physician's conduct in facilitating the woman's exercise of her reproductive freedom turn not on the viability of the fetus or on its capacity to perceive *or* on the health of the woman but, strangely, on the *physical location* of the fetus between the uterus and the vagina at the moment its development within the woman is deliberately halted—as though the fetus that is being aborted were suddenly to acquire the capacity to experience sensations of pain, or were to acquire other traits of personhood, simply by virtue of having been

moved from one point to another within the woman's body prior to completion of the abortion procedure, rather than by virtue of its own state of neurological or other development. Evidently unable to identify in any other manner the procedure they wish to outlaw, the statute's authors have thus fastened upon anatomical details that bear no relationship whatsoever even to the concern with fetal dignity or sensation that supposedly animates both the statute's title and its structure.

(1997, p. 1)

Tribe is correct that location is irrelevant to personhood, but he fails to see the implications of his insight. Conventional pro-choice belief, as expressed by Tribe, holds that infanticide is unacceptable but that abortion on demand is permissible, even late in pregnancy until the human fetus is fully outside the mother. But if location really is irrelevant, why should being born suddenly invest the child with a right to life?

One answer to this question is provided by Jose Luis Bermudez's article, "The Moral Significance of Birth." In principle, there is no difference in capacity between a fetus in utero and a baby after birth, but moral status does not hinge upon capacity but rather on the exercise of a capacity, namely the exercise of the capacity for self-awareness. Only after birth, when the newborn sees the faces of other human beings, does the baby begin to imitate their expressions, for example, tongues sticking out or mouth open wide. In order to imitate an adult, the baby expresses for the first time a primitive self-awareness. "[T]he very ability to imitate requires a rudimentary grasp of the capacity to distinguish self and other" (Bermudez 1996, p. 390). When a baby does this, it is not in Bermudez's view merely a reflex, but rather an indication of primitive self-awareness arising for the very first time. Moral significance attaches not to the *capacity* to imitate itself, which is also possessed by a late-term human fetus, but rather to the *exercise* of the capacity, which can only take place after birth (Bermudez 1996, p. 396). Once the capacity is exercised, the neonate remains primitively self-aware even when not actually imitating anyone:

If, as I have suggested, neonates can, in virtue of being born, acquire morally significant properties that cannot be possessed by full-term fetuses, then, in cases where those properties are in fact acquired, this could well confer a degree of moral significance that would make it wrong to take the life of the neonate.

(Bermudez 1996, p. 403)

Bermudez notes that his argument does not in fact entail that all neonates would enjoy moral immunity from being intentionally killed, so the argument is not that birth in itself is morally significant. Premature infants who cannot yet imitate adults would be in the same position as the fetus. In addition, full term but visually disabled infants would also be unable to exercise their capacity for imitation, since they cannot see the faces of adults. Finally, adults would in fact be able to kill as many infants as they pleased simply by making sure that they wore masks or otherwise prevented infants from seeing any human face. Indeed, one could simply blind infants at birth thereby extending indefinitely the window for killing. Such infants would never have exercised their capacity to imitate others, and so would be in the same position as the human fetus.

Is it *in principle* impossible for a late-term fetus in utero to imitate others, as Bermudez claims? It seems to be the case that twins in utero, in their many interactions, respond to and perhaps even imitate one another's actions (Piontelli 1992, ix). There is also evidence that light reaches mammals in utero (Weaver & Reppert 1989). So cases of monoamniotic twins may be able to see each other's faces and so imitate each other's expressions. If this is the case, then we have the odd conclusion that moral status depends in certain cases upon whether or not one has a monoamniotic twin sibling. Late-term abortion of such twins destroys beings with moral worth, but late-term abortion of a singlet does not. Bermudez's argument does not show that *birth* is in itself morally significant, since by nature with twinning or by technological screen in utero opportunities could be provided for such imitations of other human beings prior to birth for the fully developed human fetus.

It is also implausible to construe newborn imitation as a kind of primitive self-awareness, when neonates, indeed human beings younger than a year and a half or two years, cannot recognize themselves in a mirror (Hassoun & Kriegel 2008, p. 49). This lack of recognition suggests that there is no self-awareness, or no evidence of self-awareness, until much later than the first exercise of imitation of facial expressions. Finally, Bermudez's argument presupposes that conscious self-awareness is necessary for personhood, a view that there is reason to reject (see sections, 2.4, 2.6, 3.6, and 4.1.1).

3.5 What is Partial Birth Abortion?

Many advocates of the pro-choice view defend partial-birth abortion as legally permissible, or morally permissible, or both. Dr. Martin Haskel, in his paper "Dilation and Extraction for Late Second Trimester Abortion" delivered at the National Abortion Federation's September 1992 Risk Management Seminar, described how he performs the procedure as follows:

> With a lower [fetal] extremity in the vagina, the surgeon uses his fingers to deliver the opposite lower extremity, then the torso, the shoulders and the upper extremities. The skull lodges at the internal

cervical os. Usually there is not enough dilation for it to pass through. The fetus is oriented dorsum or spine up. At this point, the right-handed surgeon slides the fingers of the left hand along the back of the fetus and "hooks" the shoulders of the fetus with the index and ring fingers (palm down). [T]he surgeon takes a pair of blunt curved Metzenbaum scissors in the right hand. He carefully advances the tip, curved down, along the spine and under his middle finger until he feels it contact the base of the skull under the tip of his middle finger. [T]he surgeon then forces the scissors into the base of the skull or into the foramen magnum. Having safely entered the skull, he spreads the scissors to enlarge the opening. The surgeon removes the scissors and introduces a suction catheter into this hole and evacuates the skull contents. With the catheter still in place, he applies traction to the fetus, removing it completely from the patient.

(*Stenberg v. Carhart* 2000)

In *Stenberg v. Carhart*, later reversed in *Gonzales v. Carhart*, the Unites States Supreme Court affirmed a constitutional right to this procedure, partial-birth abortion, and with it affirmed the legality of the conventional pro-choice view that abortion ought to be legally permissible through all nine months of pregnancy, until the human being has been entirely removed from the mother's body. The court gave no justification why moving the head of the child just a few inches marks the crucial distinction between non-personhood and personhood; in the case of partial-birth abortion, the difference is between life and death.

In briefs to the court, some claimed that partial-birth abortion might be necessary to secure the health of the mother. However, the American Medical Association weighed in that partial-birth abortion was never medically indicated and that the procedure was more dangerous for women since it involved (partial) breach birth. The American College of Obstetricians and Gynecologists did not identify any circumstances under which partial-birth abortion would be the only way to preserve the health or life of the woman.

Another possible defense of the partial-birth abortion does not depend upon denying personhood but rather hinges on the relationship of dependency between the woman and her progeny. According to this view, the most famous formulation of which is known as the "violinist argument," the location of the fetus again becomes central in defending abortion. A consideration of this important argument will take place in chapter seven.

3.6 Reconsidering Warren's Account

Usually, justification of abortion, in its partial-birth or pre-birth form, relies on a denial of fetal personhood. While Warren's account of why infanticide is wrong but abortion is permissible is unsatisfactory from the perspective of the advocate of infanticide as well as from the perspective of a defender of fetal human life, Warren's account of personhood itself also merits fundamental reconsideration.

Patrick Lee calls into question the basis that Warren has used for developing the criteria of personhood in the first place (1996, pp. 10–11). Even if Warren is correct that the word "person" in contemporary English simply *means* a being with consciousness, reasoning, self-motivated activity, the capacity to communicate, and self-concepts, it is not clear why this is morally relevant. Why should this linguistic convention (or the concept it signifies) be taken as an *ethical* given? We can easily imagine communities in the past in which "person" (meaning the bearer of rights with inherent dignity) was used only and consistently to make reference to white, landholding men of free birth. However, the moral judgment can still be made that whatever the current use of the word "person" (or the current concept of person), we should expand its use to include others. From the opposite perspective, derogatory words (or concepts) are used widely in some communities precisely to exclude minorities from full personhood. It would not be legitimate to argue from this linguistic convention to the conclusion that such minorities lack the fullness of personhood. In sum, the meaning of words or concepts does not determine morality, so we are misguided by analyzing the "concept" of personhood to determine a resolution, one way or the other, on the question of abortion.

If Warren's criteria are accepted for the sake of argument, then depending upon how they are interpreted, some may be led to a recognition of many prenatal human beings as persons while others may decide to strip many adult human beings of personhood. If interpreted generously, several of the criteria would apply to many human beings in utero. If interpreted strictly, many human beings whose personhood has never been called into question before would suddenly be counted as non-persons lacking even the most basic rights, including the right to life.

What makes a human being a person according to at least one formulation offered by Warren is consciousness of internal and external events and the capacity to feel pain (1973, p. 263). This repeats elements from Singer's somewhat ambiguous view (section 2.4). Requiring *actual* consciousness renders us non-persons whenever we sleep. Requiring *immediately attainable* consciousness excludes those in surgery. Requiring the basic neural brain structures for consciousness (but not consciousness itself) excludes those whose brains are temporarily damaged. On the other hand, if potentiality for consciousness makes a being a person, then those sleeping, in surgery, or temporarily comatose are persons, but so also would be the normal human embryo, fetus, and newborn.

Warren's second criterion—the developed capacity to solve new and relatively complex problems—proves too much. Real problem solving doesn't begin until sometime after the age of two or perhaps even later. Hence, young children could not count as persons according to Warren's standards. And as she notes herself, neither those with dementia, the disabled, nor those suffering from Alzheimer's would count as persons either. In seeking to exclude the preborn from personhood, the handicapped, and disabled, are also stripped of rights.

Warren tries to avoid this implication by arguing that empathy for the disabled as well as for those who care and love the disabled requires that mentally handicapped human beings have full moral status (1997, p. 166). Of course, it is now unclear why empathy for the unborn and those that care for and love the unborn should not require that they have full moral status. If society as a whole becomes more hard-hearted, one could imagine empathy for the disabled and those who care for them greatly weakening. It is unreasonable and unjust to rest the moral status of handicapped human beings (or anyone else) on the emotional reaction of society.

Likewise, self-motivated activity (activity which is relatively independent of either genetic or direct external control) is present in some way in humans in utero at a very early stage. Self-initiated activity is already present at 8 to 10 weeks when human beings in utero begin to suck their thumbs and move about (though unfelt by their mothers). But if one interprets self-motivated activity in a more demanding way, then once again a whole range of human beings almost universally recognized as enjoying dignity and rights are, according to this reasoning, stripped of their personhood. The very young, the very old, the mentally handicapped, and even the addicted all lack self-motivated activity in a strong sense of autonomous, rationally informed choice.

Warren's next criterion, "the capacity to communicate, by whatever means, messages of an indefinite variety of types, that is, not just with an indefinite number of possible contents, but on indefinitely many topics," excludes from the human community of persons an indefinitely large number of human beings. It is unclear if Helen Keller, before learning sign language, or Ronald Reagan, after the onset of debilitating Alzheimer's, would count as persons.

In sum, Warren's criteria seem to legitimate much more than abortion. The senile elderly, newborns, and the mentally ill can get in the way of a "real" person's perceived freedom and happiness. On Warren's account, it would follow then that any person would be justified in killing any "potential person" whenever the existence of the potential person (e.g., a mentally handicapped teenager) got in the way of an actual person's perception of his or her health, happiness, or freedom. (Important questions should also be raised here about the authentic meaning of "happiness" and "freedom" (see Spitzer 2000)).

But there have been other definitions of personhood that avoid the difficulties of distinguishing infanticide and abortion and will include the debilitated Alzheimer's patient, the severely mentally handicapped teenager, and the coma victim. Perhaps personhood does not arise at the moment of birth but rather sometime between birth and conception. Indeed, there are a number of possibilities including sentience, brain development, viability, conscious desires, as well as others which will be explored in the next chapter.

4 Does Personhood Begin During Pregnancy?

Having examined whether personhood begins after birth, and whether it begins at birth itself, the next possibility would be that the personhood of the human fetus begins sometime between conception and birth. Between conception and birth, in terms of time and development, there are an infinite number of possible points. As Zeno pointed out, a line between two points can always be divided *ad infinitum*. So let us reflect only on some of the points along the continuum of growth that might be considered as especially noteworthy in the development of the human being in utero. Of course, there are many significant moments during gestation, so the question may arise at what point precisely does personhood begin?

4.1 What Characteristic Grants Personhood?

The most salient and often-mentioned characteristics which are held to give rise to personhood after conception and before birth include: conscious desires, viability, quickening, the ability to move spontaneously, sentience, recognizable human form, the formation of the brain, and implantation of the embryo in the uterus. Before the compelling characteristic is present, whatever that characteristic may be, abortion is fully licit. After the compelling characteristic is present, abortion would end the life of a being with moral worth. It is important to understand the relationship among these characteristics.

The story is told of a man accused of negligence because his ill-restrained dog bit someone in a park. The man's defense: "Every single time my dog is outside my house, I always keep him tightly on a leash. In addition, and I can affirm this without hesitation, my dog never goes in that park when I let him run free outdoors. Furthermore, I don't even have a dog." Just as the various elements of this man's defense are incompatible with one another, so too are the various positions with respect to fetal personhood given above incompatible with one another. If viability gives rise to personhood, then quickening, human form, and implantation do not. If the capacity to experience pain and pleasure gives rise to personhood, then spontaneous movement, brain waves, and conscious desires do not.

Thus, these theories of personhood do not together make a solid case that personhood arises somewhere between birth and conception. Rather each standard of personhood is an "independent operator" that stands or falls alone and is in competition with the other proposed standards. As such, they must each be considered in turn.

4.1.1 Conscious Desires/Interests

The interest view of personhood holds that: "if nothing at all can possibly matter to a being, then that being has no interests. Its interests therefore cannot be considered, and so the being lacks moral status" (Steinbock 1992, p. 15). It is, according to this view, a necessary condition for the right to life that a person have had conscious desires of some kind. A person is a being capable of valuing its own existence (Harris 1999, pp. 303, 307; Harris and Holm 2003, p. 116). Modifying arguments first given by Donald Marquis in his article "Why Abortion is Immoral," and the most sophisticated advocate for this view, is David Boonin who argues that killing you or me is wrong because it thwarts our desires, especially the (present, dispositional, and ideal) desire to have a future-like-ours (2003, p. 125).

The requirement of present, dispositional, and ideal desires reflects a refinement of Tooley's position explored in chapter two which connects desire and rights. The desire must be present and not future. If future desires were to count, the desire–rights analysis would also include a human embryo or fetus who will, unless killed, have desires in the future. Precisely this was what Marquis pointed to in arguing against abortion. Boonin's reason for holding that present desires give rise to the right to life is that he believes this account provides a more salient and parsimonious explanation of the impermissibility of killing in uncontroversial cases than does appeal future desires. So for Boonin, it is not future desires that make a difference to rights but present desires. This desire can be dispositional or habitual; that is, it need not be occurrent or at the moment present in consciousness, so that those who are sleeping or in comas do not lose the right to life. The desire can be ideal rather than actual, that is, it can concern what we ideally would want rather than what we in fact do want at the moment. Otherwise a suicidal, lovelorn teenager or someone whose desire not to live was created in part by false information would not have a right to life. However, until we have desires of some kind, desires whose realization requires that we not be killed, we do not have the right to life. The human fetus cannot have conscious desires prior to the point of having organized electrical activity in the cerebral cortex (Boonin 2003, p. 126). When exactly this organized electrical activity arises is itself subject to some dispute. Boonin argues that conscious desires begin at some point from 25 to 32 weeks after fertilization (2003, p. 127).

Although there is some "gray area" in determining the exact moment when this takes place, at some point between 25 and 32 weeks of gestation a human fetus begins to have conscious desires, including implicitly the desire to have a future-like-ours. Implicit desires are the necessary conditions for the fulfillment of explicit desires. The human being in the womb doesn't explicitly desire to live but since no desires can be satisfied without existing, even the simple desires of a human fetus such as the desire to hear his or her mother's voice implicitly includes the desire to live. A being with an explicit or implicit desire to live and have a future like ours thereby attains a right to life. The desire for a future like ours is deemed important since wrongdoing is viewed as frustrating our desires, in this case our desire to have a future. Until the point that desires of some kind emerge, implicitly including the desire to have a future like ours, the human fetus does not have a right to life, and so before this point feticide does not kill a being with rights. Similarly, the argument that rights presuppose interests and that interests presuppose consciousness implies that consciousness is the key to rights (Steinbock 1992, pp. 16–22). How might a defender of equal rights for all human beings respond?

The first possible way of distinguishing human beings with a right to life from humans without a right to life is by appealing to conscious desires, that is, whether they are interested in their own welfare. We've already seen two difficulties with this view. The claim that dispositional, ideal and present desires are key to the right to life in effect reiterates (in more elegant form) the ad hoc exceptions to the rule that links rights and desires made by Tooley examined earlier in section 2.3.3. Also, in section 2.4, we indicated problems with the claim that dispositional desires are morally decisive, so let us turn now to the distinction between ideal and actual desires.

The distinction between ideal and actual desires makes sense. The heartbroken suicidal teenager may not desire to live, but nevertheless has a right to life. The same is true of someone with chemical imbalances, someone working with erroneous information (e.g., the water she desires to drink is laced with a deadly poison), and a cult member who has been systematically brainwashed not to desire to live. But the distinction between ideal and actual desires corresponds to something morally important because it relies on a distinction between what appears to be good and what is actually good. As Donald Marquis put it,

> The goodness of life is not secondary to our desire for it. If this were not so, the pain of one's own premature death could be done away with merely by an appropriate alteration in the configuration of one's desires. This is absurd.

(1999, p. 53)

Desires are always desires of some good. An ideal desire is nothing other than a desire for what is actually fulfilling and good. It is the loss of what is fulfilling and good that is the problem; not the thwarting of desire. To paraphrase and slightly alter Marquis's point, it is the loss of the good of life, not the interference with the desire for that good, that constitutes the harm and hence the wrong done. And the good of life can be lost by the lovelorn teenager, the brainwashed cult follower, and the human fetus alike.

A critic might agree that the loss of life is the harm that is endured by the human being in utero and not simply the interference with desires, but that it is a different question than whether the human being has a right not to be harmed in this way. One could hold that a plant is harmed if you fail to water it, but also hold that the plant has no right to be watered. Similarly, one could concede that the human fetus at all stages of development is harmed by the loss of life, but that this harm only matters morally when the human fetus has some actual desires.

This chapter is not trying to establish that every human being should be respected; that is the task for the next chapter. Rather, it is attempting to show that various other accounts of why some human beings but not all human beings have rights are mistaken. The human being in utero who is killed is harmed by losing life not simply by having various desires thwarted, but whether or not all human beings have rights not to be intentionally killed is still at issue. The point is simply that emphasis on desire as the key element of having rights is misplaced.

Moreover, one can imagine beings that are indisputably persons but would be excluded by Boonin's understanding of the right to life. Consider alien, angelic, or divine persons who, given their vast differences from our fragile human physiology, have nothing that corresponds to what we experience as desire. Nor is it difficult to imagine alien, angelic, or divine persons whose experiences of time are so different from our own that they do not experience past, present, and future as we do and so have no present dispositional desires for a future like ours. Even among human persons, there are those such as Buddhists who believe that the extinguishing of all desire is possible. If a human being achieved this goal, then this human being would have achieved Nirvana from a Buddhist perspective, but from Boonin's perspective would thereby no longer have a right to life, since such a human being, the Buddhist Master, would not have a desire for the future. Christians, Jews, and Muslims also hold that human beings in heaven cease having desires, since desires indicate a lack of perfection incompatible with the fullness of heavenly joy.

Consider another case. A 25-year-old contractor named Phineas Gage, Jr. walks up a flight of stairs holding a nail gun, slips on a stray bit of wood, and fires a nail straight into his skull. Astonishingly, Phineas does not die. Surgeons carefully remove the nail from his skull, and after a period of recovery, Phineas leaves the hospital. He continues life much as before with only one important difference. Phineas notices that he no longer desires anything. It so happens that the nail damaged exactly the part of his brain that controls feelings of desire. So although he is fully rational, although he can speak, calculate, and otherwise live as before the nail entered his brain, he no longer has any desires of any kind. Poor Phineas clearly suffers a neurological pathology, but it is absurd to claim that Phineas would also no longer be a being with a right to live.

Consider another case. A mad scientist discovers the neural pathways that allow human beings to experience desire. She also discovers a drug, which she names Nirvana Now, which permanently blocks the chemical reactions in the brain that are necessary for anyone to have desires. Some people take the drug that permanently blocks their desires. It becomes popular among aspiring Buddhist masters as a chemical route to what they had sought through religious practice. The people who take Nirvana Now, let's call one of them Lisa, are exactly like us in every respect, but they no longer have any desires whatsoever. It is reasonable to say that we can kill them at will?

Might Phineas and Lisa have an ideal desire to live, since their current condition of lacking desire arises from a pathology of some kind? No, says Boonin, "a particular ideal desire can meaningfully be attributed only to someone who has at least some other actual desires" (2003, p. 80). This condition also excludes Lisa, the Buddhist master, and the heavenly persons mentioned earlier. Put in terms of the interest view of dignity, Phineas no longer takes an interest in his own well-being, so he no longer has moral status. As in the case of space aliens (Warren) and talking cats (Tooley), whether Phineas, angels, heavenly persons, or Buddhist masters actually exist is not relevant. However, if they did exist, they would obviously and uncontroversially be persons, and if they are persons, the conscious desires or interest account is clearly mistaken.

Paradoxically, for the conscious desires account of personhood, it is a lack of perfection, the negation of a good quality rather than its possession that justifies the claim that the being in question should be respected. Beings of higher perfection (angels, heavenly persons, Buddhist masters), possessing superior qualities, end up deserving less respect than those of lower perfection (regular human beings) who can only desire to have such superior qualities. If such lower beings ever got that which they desired, the end of desire (either by enjoying the sought good perfectly or by extinguishing desire), they would no longer be worthy of moral respect.

Of course, if a being did not desire to continue to live (since the being fully enjoys continuous life without possibility of its loss), then it would seem that the right to life would be otiose. Such a being cannot be killed, and so such a being does not need (and therefore) does not have a right to life.

However, it is entirely possible to violate someone's moral rights without inflicting any actual damage upon them. Attempted assault, rape, or murder is wrong even if such an attempt did not and could not have succeeded. If Superwoman existed, no one would be able to rape her. But a man who attempted to rape her would wrong her nonetheless. If wearing a bulletproof vest, the President of the United States may be in a certain respect invulnerable, but the would-be assassin who shoots the Commander-in-Chief in the chest has wronged the President nonetheless. Thus, the right to life of a being who enjoys continuous life without possibility of loss could still be violated, by an attempted murder. One's rights include a protection not only against loss of a good you enjoy, but against another attempting to undermine your good.

A critic might object that if a being (angel, Phineas, Lisa, or alien) does not have desires then it is not clear that they have a future like ours. If they don't have a future like ours, then we cannot ground their right to live in this characteristic.

But even though such beings would lack desires (of a future good), they nevertheless could have enjoyment (of a present good). If they also have a future, then they would also have a future like ours, possibly filled with enjoyments. Would they not then also desire to have this future? We certainly do. However, it is possible that such creatures do not have such desires if, for example, their sense of time is different than ours. Even for us, to be fully immersed in a currently enjoyed good sometimes virtually suspends the sense of time passing or concern for the future. Angels or aliens may have this sense to a maximally heightened degree. Poor Phineas had that part of his brain which concerns anticipating future events also damaged so that he does not have actual desires for the future.

In any case, another important problem can be raised about the conscious desires argument. If one believes in "certain inalienable rights, that among these are life, liberty and the pursuit of happiness" as it is put in the *Declaration of Independence* (1776), then the link between desires and rights is not as Boonin portrays it. Inalienable rights are rights that a person cannot waive or give up regardless of their desires. Alienable rights, on the other hand, are rights that depend on the desires of the person and so one can waive such rights. For instance, the right you have to your watch is an alienable right, and so you can give up your claim to this watch and give it to another as a gift without violating anyone's rights.

On the other hand, one's desires, whatever they may be, have no bearing on inalienable rights. A common example of an inalienable right is the right to liberty. Even if a person desires to be a slave, and another person desires to be a slave master, if the right to liberty is inalienable, then slavery violates the right to liberty. Inalienable rights can only be made void by legitimate public authority in the case of just punishment. So, if liberty is an inalienable right, then only just punishment for criminal wrongdoing could make void that right. Since the right to life is a necessary condition for the right to liberty, if the right to liberty is an inalienable right, the right to life would also be inalienable. If the right to life is inalienable, as most theorists of human rights have held, then Boonin's account of why killing is wrong must be rejected because one's right to life does not depend in any way on one's (present, dispositional, ideal) desires. Most critics of abortion also hold that the right to life is inalienable. So, at least in one important respect, Boonin has failed in his attempt to show that "the moral case against abortion can be shown to be unsuccessful on terms that critics of abortion can, and already do, accept" (2003, p. 2).

Perhaps the case of permanently comatose adults indicates that the right to life is not an inalienable right. Many people think that a permanently comatose adult does not have the same right to life as healthy adults since it is morally permissible to no longer continue to support such human beings with life-saving medical treatments. We can stop providing medical care to people in permanent comas which results in their deaths, so such people do not share an equal right to life with temporarily comatose human persons.

Here, it is important to understand more precisely what is meant by the right to life. Your right to life is the duty of other people not to kill you intentionally. It is not the duty of other people to do whatever it takes to keep you alive. As noted earlier (section 2.5), we can affirm the basic equal moral worth of all human beings without also affirming the basic worth of all medical treatments. Whether a given medical treatment is a good idea to administer depends upon the likely burdens and benefits of that treatment. The likely burdens and benefits of a given treatment will vary from patient to patient, depending upon the particularities to the situation and wider context. In some cases, a given treatment will be viewed by the patient or the patient's surrogate as more burdensome than beneficial, and such a treatment can be removed or not be started without a denial of the fundamental equality of the patient with all other human beings. The removal of medical treatments in such contexts is not a violation of the patient's right to live.

Even if killing is wrong because it eliminates future experiences that we have a present dispositional desire to preserve, and even if this is the best account of why killing is wrong, the conscious desires account of personhood requires that this be the only reason why killing is wrong. But this is unreasonable. An act is often wrong for a number of reasons at once. For example, a nasty caricature of a black woman might be cruel, racist, and sexist. There are myriad possible reasons to believe killing is wrong. For instance, killing takes away your present good, the good of life. Killing undermines your bodily well-being. Killing takes away your freedom. If killing is wrong for one of these reasons, or if killing is wrong for any other reason unconnected with my or your (present, dispositional, ideal) desires (e.g., divine command, societal cohesion, rule-utilitarianism, Rawls's maximin principle, contractarianism), then the suggested criterion for establishing the right to life fails. The conscious desires account of personhood requires not just that killing is wrong because it takes away your or my (present, dispositional, and ideal) desires for a future. The conscious desires account of personhood requires that killing is wrong only for this reason. In other words, for the conscious desires argument to work, it is also necessary that all other actual and possible accounts of the impermissibility of killing unrelated to desire are mistaken. Of course, this has not been demonstrated by advocates of the desire account, nor does demonstrating it seem at all likely. Indeed, one would have to refute Kant, Aristotle, Mill, and virtually every other philosopher who has given an account of the impermissibility of killing in order for this version of personhood to work.

However, let's assume for the sake of argument that killing is wrong because and only because it thwarts a human being's present desires for a future. It is important to note that the desires of human beings for various ends, including life, vary considerably, and so it would seem that the wrongness of acting against someone's desires would vary considerably too. After all, if what is wrong with some act is that it contradicts someone's desires, then it would seem to follow that the more someone desires something, the more wrong it would be to contradict the person's desire. If you steal my favorite heirloom given to me by my grandfather on his deathbed, you have wronged me more than if you steal my can of Diet Pepsi. As Boonin himself notes, "It is in general *prima facie* wrong to act in ways that frustrate the desires of others, and in general more seriously *prima facie* wrong to act in ways that frustrate their stronger desires" (2003, p. 67). This makes sense with property rights because property clearly has different values for the person whose rights are violated. It is more wrong to steal $10,000 than $10, and more wrong to steal from a poor widow than from Bill Gates.

But when one considers the value of human persons, it is a truism to affirm their fundamental equality. We generally do not hold some murders to be "better" murders than others. They are all wrong and wrong for the same reason(s); and the concept of equal rights leads us to hold they are equally wrong. One might object that killing a parent who cares for his or her three young children is worse than killing a person without dependent children. But the truth of this does not undermine the equality of persons, the idea which leads one to hold that all murder is equally bad considered in itself, even if circumstances may make some murders worse in terms of consequences for others. Thus, the murder of a parent is wrong both because it is murder, which is wrong for whatever reason(s), and in addition because it deprives the young children of someone upon whom they depend. This additional aspect of wrongness could be in play in non-murderous situations, such as kidnapping or permanently and seriously injuring the parent. The murder of the person who does not have dependent children is equally wrong and considered as murder. If human persons have equal rights, then murdering human persons is equally wrong whether the person is rich or poor, black or white, male or female.

Such equality is not found in people's desires. Just as there is wide diversity in human desires generally, it is undoubtedly true that people do not have equal desires to live. As Victor Frankl noted in his book *Man's Search for Meaning*, in Nazi concentration camps some people ended their own lives after just a few days, while others were determined to live in spite of all obstacles. Even in less extreme circumstances, it is obvious that people value their lives differently. Some people absolutely minimize all risks to bodily safety; other people take great risks with their lives; still other people take their own lives. It would follow from the account of wrongfulness given by Boonin that killing those who didn't want to live wasn't wrong at all, killing those who wanted to live a little bit was worse, and killing those who really wanted to live was the worst of all. But this would mean that the victims in the camp, indeed persons in general, do not enjoy fundamentally equal rights to life—which, of course, is problematic if one wants to affirm the fundamental equality of all persons. If Boonin's argument was correct, it would show not only that the human fetus does not have the same right to life as you or I, but also that you and I don't have the same right to life. Indeed, since no two human persons have exactly the same desire to live, so no two human persons have equal rights to life. Since life is necessary to exercise any other right, if Boonin's account is correct, equal rights are an illusion.

One retort to this critique would be that the differences of desires among human beings are differences of *actual* desires rather than differences with respect to *ideal* desires. Our actual desires to live do differ radically, but perhaps our ideal desires to live do not differ radically but are exactly the same, giving rise to equal rights to life.

Given what we know about desires, it is unlikely that even ideal desires are *exactly* the same for *all* human persons. But let's assume for the sake of argument that they are. What would explain the fact that the ideal desires to live of human beings are exactly the same? It would seem plausible to say that they are the same because they are desires for the very same good—the good of life. But if the ideal desires account ultimately rests on the foundation of the good of life—a good which is shared equally by the human fetus, the human newborn, and the human adult—then we no longer have grounds for excluding certain human beings from consideration as persons.

Another retort to this critique would be to distinguish between harm and impermissibility. I cause more harm by stealing $50,000 than by stealing $50; I cause more harm by stealing from a poor person than by stealing from a rich person. The harm caused may be greater or lesser. However,

I have no more right to steal $50 than to steal $50,000. In each case, I have no right whatsoever to steal, and therefore the property owners have equal rights to retain their property. In the same way, it does more harm (normally) to kill a young person than an old person, and more harm to kill a person who greatly desires to live than a person who is weary of life. Although the amount of harm differs in various kinds of killing, all these persons have an equal right to life because others have no right to kill them. Since in all cases of illicit killing, the killer has no right to kill, one might also say that in such cases the victims had equal rights to live.

This objection fails in part because it proves too much. It proves not only that all people have an equal right to life, but it proves that all rights whatsoever are equal, for in every case of rights violation, the other person had no right to violate it. I have no right to kill you and no right to steal $5 from you, so the right to life and the right to keep the $5 are equal rights. But if all rights are equal, this causes a difficulty because it often happens that rights conflict with one another. Your right to control your body (say, by punching your fist) may conflict with my right to bodily integrity (not to have my face bludgeoned by blows). But not all rights are in fact equal, for my right to bodily integrity (presumably) takes precedence over your right to move your fists where you would like. Everyone has an equal right to life, but all rights whatsoever are not equal as the harm/permissibility objection contends in trying to secure an equal right to life for everyone. Indeed, some rights take precedent over others, and since the previous arguments lead to the conclusion that all rights are equal (a view rejected, quite sensibly, by Boonin (2003, p. 137)), it cannot be maintained.

However, let's assume that all these critiques of the conscious desires argument for personhood are mistaken. Let's assume that all persons must have desires for a future and that killing is wrong only because it thwarts our present desire to have a future and that the argument about equal rights doesn't succeed or isn't important. Nevertheless, the conscious desires argument for personhood still fails because it proves too much. Each year in the United States alone, nearly half a million babies, more than 10% of births, are born prematurely. According to the 2002 National Vital Statistics report, more than 28,895 babies were born in the United States before 28 weeks and more than 48,624 babies were born between 28 and 31 weeks during the year 2000 alone. If human beings do not have the desires which grant them a right to life until 32 weeks following conception, then more than 77,000 babies born during a single year in the United States alone would not be persons.

Could we draw the line earlier still at say 20 weeks? Citing the work of others (Morowitz & Terfil 1992), Boonin states that, "Adopting this very conservative estimate [of personhood beginning at 20 weeks] seems advisable given our lack of more definitive knowledge" (2003, p. 128). The idea seems to be that when definitive knowledge is lacking, one should err on the side of granting rights. But it is not at all clear why definitive knowledge is not present, if it is also true that, "there is no evidence to suggest that this [conscious desire] occurs prior to approximately the 25th week of gestation, and ample evidence to suggest that it does begin to occur sometime between the 25th and 32nd week" (Boonin 2003, p. 115). If there is no evidence that the line should be at 20 weeks and ample evidence that the line should not be at 20 weeks (but rather between the 25th and 32nd week), then it seems reasonable to say we have definitive knowledge that the line is not at 20 weeks. If our standards for "definitive knowledge" are higher still, approaching absolute certainty, then it is hard to see why we should not grant the right to life to the human being in utero from conception onward, if protection of human life is the default position when lacking definitive knowledge. After all, it would be hard to claim near absolute certainty about virtually anything, let alone something as controversial as the beginnings of human personhood.

Even if the line were drawn at 20 weeks, it is highly likely in the future that some newborns would still not count as persons according to this theory. Some rare, lucky newborns have survived at 21 weeks, and there is no reason to think that they will not survive earlier and earlier as technology progresses. For Boonin, this would appear to be a problem since he criticizes other theories for being unable to account for the presumed wrongfulness of infanticide (2003, p. 125).

In fact, Boonin's account cannot secure the right to life of even full term infants. Boonin is correct that full term infants, as well as the human fetus at a certain stage of development, can experience pain and may respond "positively" to certain stimuli such as hearing the mother's voice or being fed, and he concludes from this that a newborn has actual desires (2003, p. 83).

However, it does not follow from that fact that newborns enjoy certain sensations that they desire these sensations. A being may enjoy experiencing pleasure and may not enjoy experiencing pain, but it does not yet follow that the being desires pleasure or does not desire pain. In other words, merely enjoying sensations is not sufficient for having desires. Desiring involves more than simply experiencing a series of positive and negative sensations. To desire is to envision that some possibility may be or not be, and then, following this judgment, to prefer that some possibility is or is not realized. To desire, in other words, requires both belief and judgment. At the least, we desire something that we believe we do not yet enjoy. If we believe we already enjoy something we do not desire it (although we may desire to continue enjoying it). Unless suffering from gross misunderstanding, human beings do not desire to be members of the species *Homo sapiens*. So, desires involve a modicum of belief. In addition, to desire involves a judgment that it would be good to have whatever is not yet had. We only desire what is, in our opinion, good, fulfilling, and perfecting of ourselves. To desire, in other words, requires a belief (that something is not the case), and judgment (that this same something is worth having).

Many philosophers hold that beings without language do not, properly speaking, have beliefs (Malcolm 1977; Davidson 1984; Stich 1983). If they are correct, and if desires presuppose beliefs, then Boonin's account would not accord a human being the right to life until months after birth when a child first learns to speak. This is much too late, even for advocates of infanticide such as Peter Singer and Michael Tooley.

A critic could respond that the infant, even if he or she does not have desires properly speaking, surely has preferences. For example, a baby prefers to nurse when hungry than be ignored. We can base a right to live then on these minimal preferences, preferences that would not be had by any human being prior to a certain stage of brain development.

However, to have preferences is to compare different states of affairs through acts of memory or imagination or both, *and* to make a judgment of one over the other. I prefer strawberry to chocolate ice cream, but I could not do this unless I had some memory of the taste of both flavors and judge strawberry as superior. There is no evidence of which I am aware that a newborn infant has acts of memory or imagination. Newborns also cannot make judgments, so infants do not have preferences—though they may enjoy or not enjoy certain experiences.

However, even if one had a more modest account of what is required to have a desire or preference, even if we hold that animals such as squirrels have beliefs and desires (MacIntyre 1999), Boonin's view that human beings have desires 32 weeks following conception may still run into difficulties. A squirrel may be said to desire the nut, since (1) the squirrel realizes that it does not yet have the nut and (2) judges that the nut, and not say the rock which it also does not have, would be good for it. However, there is no evidence that the healthy full term newborn has the requisite intellectual powers of belief and judgment exercised by the squirrel. The newborn experiences pain in being hungry, and then satisfaction in nursing, but these alternating experiences do not yet amount to desire. The healthy newborn does not have beliefs nor can the infant make judgments that something would be good to have. Only well after birth does a human child have the requisite powers of belief and judgment to have actual desires akin even to a squirrel's, so given the conscious desires account healthy full term newborns would not have moral immunity from infanticide. If belief and judgment are not necessary for moral worth, if simply experiencing pleasure and pain is sufficient for interests of some kind (Steinbock 1992, pp. 23, 57–58), then, in effect, the conscious desires account has been abandoned in favor of a version of the sentience model of moral worth and rights—a version which will be treated below in section 4.1.4.

4.1.2 Viability

Occurring before the onset of fetal conscious experience, viability is an influential way to distinguish mere humans from persons. As used by the U.S. Supreme Court in *Roe v. Wade*, viability refers to the point when the human being in utero is "potentially able to live outside the mother's womb, albeit with artificial aid." This U.S. Supreme Court decision held that viability is an important distinguishing mark between human fetuses that deserve some protection under the law and those that do not. The ability to survive outside the womb marks the junction where the state could begin to outlaw abortion in some limited circumstance so long as abortion otherwise remained permissible to preserve the life and health of the mother. Even though restriction of feticide following viability was allowed in principle, one should not ignore the important qualification that was made to this ruling about maternal health. Unlike most Western countries, legalized abortion in the United States was extended through all nine months of pregnancy by the U.S. Supreme Court decision *Doe v. Bolton*, a companion decision issued on the same day as *Roe*. *Doe* defined the "health" of the mother in a broad manner that would include mental health, family situation, and other factors understood comprehensively. In other words, the desire not to have a baby could count as a "health" reason under this decision.

In any case, the U. S. Supreme Court in the *Roe* decision singled out viability as an important feature in connection with the personhood of the human fetus. Why is viability so important? Viability marks the moment at which the fetus has the capability of living outside the womb, and so it also marks the beginning of an independent existence in terms of human rights. One could easily modify this view slightly and say this moment is not only a compelling moment when certain kinds of restriction on abortion could be justified in some circumstances but also the defining moment when a human being becomes a person. If this analysis is accepted, then abortion after viability would be killing an innocent human person but abortion before viability would not be. How might an advocate of equal rights for all human beings respond?

The court's reasoning in *Roe v. Wade* for holding that viability is a compelling point for the state to take legal interest in the human fetus (presumably because the fetus then has some moral worth) is stated only once and very briefly, "With respect to the State's important and legitimate interest in potential life, the 'compelling' point is at viability. This is so because the fetus then presumably has the capability of meaningful life outside the mother's womb" (*Roe v. Wade* 1973). But this justification, aside from the word "meaningful," is simply a restatement of the definition of viability. Viability is achieved when the fetus has the capacity to live outside the mother's womb, and this is important, we are told, because it is when the fetus has the capacity to survive outside the mother's womb. This circular reasoning does not justify granting viability any significance.

Michael Tooley, whose defense of infanticide was discussed in the second chapter, holds, in fact, that there are reasons to reject viability as a way to distinguish mere humans from persons (1972, p. 51). If the human fetus could learn a language, and use of language is a sufficient condition of personhood, then the human being in utero who speaks would be a person. Just imagine if at an ultrasound appointment, we not only saw the movement of the human being in utero but also heard a voice, asking mom perhaps to eat more zucchini and avoid the salsa, or strenuously objecting to being named "Brandi." Physiological dependency has no relationship to personhood.

Tooley also points out that conjoined or "Siamese" twins sometimes depend on one another for life and yet both are considered persons. Consider the case of the conjoined twins known by the pseudonyms "Jodie" and "Mary." Born in Manchester, England on August 8, 2000, Mary and Jodie's appearance was so unusual and their disabilities so severe that several doctors had to excuse themselves from giving care to the twins. Jodie and Mary were joined at the lower abdomen and shared a spine. Though both twins had nearly a full complement of organs, Jodie's heart and lungs maintained both of their lives since Mary's were not sufficiently developed to pump oxygenated blood. Doctors predicted that Jodie's circulatory system would give out in a matter of weeks under the strain of supporting both girls. Judges, doctors, and ethicists considered a decision to rival Solomon's: Should one twin be sacrificed in order to save the other or should both be allowed to perish? Although a British Court ordered them separated, there was no clear consensus about how to answer this question. No one, however, claimed that Mary was not really a person since her life was entirely dependent on her sister's. In fact, a British court mentioned the issue of whether Mary's dependence on Jodie robbed her of personhood only to dismiss the contention in the most caustic terms. Even though Mary was not viable independent of Jodie, she was still a person.

Other philosophers have rejected viability as a standard for differentiating persons from mere humans because studies have shown that African fetuses become viable before Latino fetuses and Latino fetuses before Caucasian fetuses (Alexander et al. 2003). Female fetuses become viable before male fetuses, and fetuses in wealthy countries with access to advanced health care become viable before fetuses in poor countries without such access. However, differences of race, sex, and affluence should have absolutely no bearing on personhood.

Viability also leads to paradoxical results—that the very same being in utero may go back and forth numerous times, perhaps every day, between being a person with a right to life and a mere human fetus who can be killed at will. Peter Singer writes:

Suppose that a woman who is twenty-five weeks pregnant is living in Melbourne, a city with excellent intensive care units for premature babies, but she then travels to a remote part of the desert west of Alice Springs, three days from the nearest airstrip. Are we to believe that the fetus inside her was a living human being when she was in Melbourne, but not when she was in the desert? What happened to it, then? Did it die? Did it cease to be human? Merely asking these questions shows how untenable it is to make the start of a new human life dependent upon viability.

(1994, p. 102)

A human fetus in a flight attendant 25 weeks pregnant would be a person on the ground and then cease being a person with each flight. The fact that the technology is available at a hospital somewhere on the ground to maintain the life of the fetus does not change the fact that the flying fetus is not, in fact, viable.

One could argue that even if not actually viable during flight, such humans in utero are capable of being viable because the technology exists somewhere (even if not in mid-flight) that could keep them alive. However, such a technologically dependent standard may turn out to be an unreliable means of justifying abortion. Indeed, with the advance of technology, viability may one day be possible throughout pregnancy. As former U.S. Supreme Court Justice Sandra Day O'Connor pointed out, *Roe* is on a collision course with itself. Within recent memory, the limit of viability was considered to be at 30 weeks. In 2007, baby Amillia Taylor pushed the barrier of viability to 21 weeks. If science continues to progress at this rate, then it is possible that within the lifetimes of college students today the human fetus will be viable outside the womb from very early in pregnancy. Of course, medical advances are not locked on to a timeline, so breakthroughs might speed this process up considerably. It is nonsensical to believe that technology determines who is and is not a person, since technology bears no necessary relationship to personhood. Technology may indeed determine who lives or dies. In the future, perhaps the injuries that now bring about irreversible brain death could be treated so that the person does not die from what now are lethal injuries. But such breakthroughs in sustaining human life do not differ in kind from penicillin that saved those who previously would have been doomed to death. Writing prior to the survival of baby Amillia Taylor at 21 weeks, Julian Savulescu wrote,

Viability is dependent on the state of technology. Over the last 20 years, it has dropped from 28 weeks to 24 weeks. So, if the fetus's right not to be killed is determined by viability, a fetus has a right not to be killed at 24 weeks now, but it did not have this right 20 years ago. Indeed, whether a fetus has a right to life will depend on its gestation, the extent of its abnormalities, the country and even the centre in which it is born. But why should our rights depend on these contingencies? A person with incurable cancer still has a right to life even if technology cannot save her.

(2001, p. 168)

So, as Tooley and Singer suggest, viability is a very poor way to distinguish persons from mere humans.

4.1.3 Quickening/Fetal Movement

Quickening is another possible way to mark the distinction between human non-persons and human persons. The first movements of the human being in the womb felt by the mother has, in law and in moral reflection, been held to be a moment when the human fetus acquires the stature of full or at least partial personhood. Why is quickening the critical point?

One argument holds that quickening is important because quickening indicates the existence of a living being within the mother. If movement is one of the essential principles of life, then the movement of something on its own indicates that the being in question is alive. Hence, only when the human fetus can generate its own movement does it begin to have life and moral importance. At quickening, the mother first recognizes the movement of fetal life within her and so at this point the human fetus becomes a person. Therefore, feticide before quickening would be permissible, but abortion after quickening might be impermissible.

A second argument suggests that prior to quickening the human fetus is held to be simply a part of the mother. After quickening the human being in utero is independent of the mother as is shown by its own independently generated movements. If the human embryo or human fetus is simply a part of the women's body, then it might be likened to an appendix, or tonsils, or perhaps a tumor. One can hardly object to the removal of such things, or to other alterations of one's own body. If the fetus is simply a part of the mother's body, then abortion belongs among other voluntary alterations of the human body such as breast augmentation, breast reduction, capping teeth, nose jobs, tummy tucks, stapling the stomach, laser eye surgery, and removal of polyps. Perhaps there might be circumstantial grounds to oppose these procedures. Consider a parent who failed to feed his or her children in order to save money for Botox injections to reduce wrinkles. Nothing is wrong in itself about getting such injections, but it would not be right to use money in that way if doing so would lead to the parent's children starving. However, considered in themselves, controlling, manipulating, or altering one's own body does not seem in general to be matters of great moral concern though even these may be matters for concern in some situations. So if it turns out that the human embryo/fetus is simply a part of the woman's body, say similar to her appendix, then a moral objection to abortion in itself fails. Quickening has been seen as the moment in which this human fetus indicates its independence from the mother, so quickening is the moment when the human fetus gains personhood.

These same two arguments could be altered slightly in favor of holding that self-initiated fetal movement, even if not felt by the mother, marks the beginning of personhood for the prenatal human being. Ultrasound indicates that fetal movement can take place around seven weeks following conception. So if fetal movement is essential for indicating the existence of a living being which has an existence in some sense independent from the mother, this transition can be shown to take place even before any movement is experienced by the mother. So if movement is essential for personhood, then before fetal movement, the human being in utero is not a person; but after self-initiated movement the human being in utero gains personhood.

A difficulty with this view is that it is hard to reconcile with widely held intuitions about which beings deserve respect. Paralyzed adults may not move but would seem to still have a right to life (Tooley, 1972, p. 53); on the other hand, insects and machines may move but presumably do not have a right to life. Moreover, if simple movement qualified a being as having a right not to be killed then the human fetus would have a right to life months before birth.

Two arguments were given in favor of quickening as a significant marker in the transition from mere humanity to personhood. It was said that prior to quickening the human fetus is simply a part of the mother, and quickening is important because independently generated movements show clearly that the human being in utero is separate from the mother. Although mothers do not sense this movement until between 16 and 20 weeks, ultrasound technology reveals fetal movement as early as seven or eight weeks. So if the independent movement of the fetus is the essential thing, and this movement begins at seven or eight weeks, then this is the time when one can clearly differentiate the mother from the fetus, not quickening.

The same point can be made about the second argument for the importance of quickening, which holds that since movement is one of the essential principles of life, then the movement of something on its own indicates that the being in question is a living being not identical with its mother. Hence, only when the human fetus can generate its own movement does it begin to have moral importance. But since this movement takes place well before it is sensed by the mother, quickening is not important but rather the beginning of fetal movement at seven or eight weeks.

Both the arguments in favor of quickening, or in modified form in favor of fetal movement as the sign of personhood, presuppose that personhood arises from not being a part of the mother. If the fetus can move, then it has its own life and it is not simply part of the mother. And if the fetus is not simply part of the mother, then the human being in utero is his or her own person.

But the view that the human fetus is simply part of the mother, even before fetal movement at seven or eight weeks, faces some serious objections. It often happens that the human fetus has a different blood type than the mother, has a different eye color than the mother, or has a different sex than the mother. Barring cloning, the human fetus always has a different genetic code than the mother, and even with cloning the fetus would not be exactly identical to the mother for even monozygotic twins have different fingerprints. The mother and a clone would also differ in age and physical development. These facts indicate that the human fetus is not just another part of the mother.

This same truth is seen by the absurdities that arise if one supposes that the fetus is simply part of the mother. If the fetus is simply part of the mother, then one has to hold bizarre views such as that pregnant women have four feet, four hands, and two heads, and in case of twins, that pregnant women have three heads. It would follow that when pregnant with a male offspring, a women has a penis.

Even apart from these bizarre counterfactuals, to be within something or someone does not make one a part of something or someone. *In vitro* fertilization (IVF) indicates this quite clearly. A "test tube" baby is not part of the Petri dish, even though at the beginning of life such human beings reside within a Petri dish. IVF makes clear that the human fetus is not simply part of the mother in another way. In July 2002, the BBC reported the birth of twin black babies to a white couple. After creation outside the womb in a Petri dish, a lab mix-up led to a women giving birth to children not biologically related to her. In this case, a woman with no African lineage whatsoever gave birth to babies with a black biological father and black biological mother. Of course, the twins did not suddenly become Caucasian simply because they were growing within a white mother nor was the mother suddenly black because of the twins. Likewise, if a black woman nourished twins in utero conceived by IVF from the gametes of white parents, the children born would be white. Quite clearly, human beings in utero are separate human beings from their mothers.

Finally, it can also happen that the human fetus dies and the mother lives independently for many years or that the mother dies but the human being who was in utero at the time of his or her mother's death lives on independently for many years. Consider for example the case of Trisha Marshall and her son Darious (Singer 1994, pp. 9–11). On April 19, 1993, Trisha attacked a man with a meat cleaver, and he responded by shooting her in the head and on April 21 she was declared brain dead. She was also 17 weeks pregnant. At the insistence of her boyfriend as well as her parents, a respirator helped her maintain some bodily functions including maintaining Darious developing insider her. On August 3, 1993, three and a half months after his mother was declared brain dead, Darious was born via caesarean birth, a healthy and, according to a doctor at the hospital, "cute" baby boy. Of course, one might say that this case is very good evidence that higher brain "death" is not really death but only severe head trauma to a person who continues to live. But one could easily change the details of this case and come to a similar insight. If a late-term pregnant woman is beheaded (no doubt about death there), the fetus could be removed from the corpse and live. The death of the mother is not the death of the fetus; the death of the fetus is not the death of the mother. This fact shows that mother and offspring are two different human beings with independent lives. Since the human fetus is not simply a part of the mother, the arguments based on this belief such as those in favor of the moral significance of quickening or unfelt fetal movement are not sound.

4.1.4 *Sentience*

According to some philosophers, it is with sentience, the capacity to suffer pain or enjoy pleasure, that a being begins to have interests; and if one links interests and rights, sentience would mark the beginning of the right to life. According to this view, as soon as a human being in utero develops the capacity to feel pleasure or suffer pain, the human fetus would begin to have interests that should count equally with every other sentient being's interests. Indeed, if interests give rise to rights, then at this point the human fetus could acquire rights, including the right to life. On this view, the rights of the human fetus, including the right to life, would arise at the same time as a capacity for pain and pleasure developed (Sumner 1981).

So when does the human fetus attain the capacity to experience pleasure and pain? Ronald Green believes that sentience arises perhaps 30–35 weeks after conception, just a few weeks before full term birth. However, he concedes that after the formation of the forebrain, midbrain, and hindbrain, sentience cannot be ruled out (Green 2001, p. 42). Human sentience requires a brain, and at five weeks following conception, the fetus develops a deeply creased and convoluted cerebral cortex. Given that the fetus does have a functioning brain, and reacts to stimuli of all sorts within the first trimester of pregnancy, there is reason to believe that sentience, the capacity to feel, begins fairly early, in the first trimester of pregnancy by the seventh week (Oderberg 2000, pp. 6–8).

Although there are debates about when the human fetus becomes sentient, the importance of sentience is underscored by any view that links sentience with interests and interests with rights. According to the sentience account, once sentience begins, whether this is at ten weeks or 36 weeks, then the mere human being of the fetus becomes a human person with a right to life.

A critic of the view that sentience confers rights might question why experiencing pleasure and pain is so important to having rights. Why should a being's moral value depend upon sentience, its ability to experience pleasure and pain? Peter Singer writes:

> The most obvious reason for valuing the life of a being capable of experiencing pleasure and pain is the pleasure it can experience. If we value our own pleasures—like the pleasures of eating, of sex, of running at full speed, and of swimming on a hot day—then the universal aspect of ethical judgment requires us to extend our positive evaluation of our own experience of these pleasures to similar experiences of all who can experience them. But death is the end of all pleasurable experiences. Thus the fact that a being will experience pleasure in the future is reason for saying that it would be wrong to kill them.
>
> (2000, p. 139)

But the typical human fetus, unless terminated, is quite obviously a being that will experience pleasure in the future, so if Singer's analysis is correct, then he has provided grounds for opposing both abortion throughout pregnancy and infanticide.

One could shore up this difficulty with the sentience argument by saying that it is not future sentience that matters but current sentience. A being who actually and presently experiences or can experience pleasure and pain has moral standing, but a being who does not currently experience pleasure or pain does not. But this adjustment thereby also excludes those who are in surgery under anesthesia or in a temporary coma. Repeated surgeries or repeated comas raise, once again, the episodic problem.

We could assume that the brain structure required for sentience is what really counts, not actually being sentient or potentially being sentient. But on this account, one wonders why this one necessary condition for sentience—neural brain structure—is chosen rather than some other necessary condition for sentience, say, actually being conscious or being alive or the genetic basis for sentience.

Let's assume these difficulties with the argument from sentience to moral worth can be overcome. Although sentience is often seen as a morally significant moment in the development of the preborn human being, it is also a quality believed to be shared by numerous beings who are clearly not persons such as leeches, locusts, and wasps. But surely we don't do wrong by using pesticide on a wasp, since sentience does not give rise to the right to life.

However, in response, a defender of abortion might note that not all sentient beings are *equally* sentient, so as to avoid according equal rights to insects. According to this version of the sentience argument, early abortion is morally unproblematic because the early human fetus is not yet sentient. But this makes room for the intuition that the later in pregnancy feticide takes place the more problematic it is since human sentience grows as pregnancy progresses. Differences in sentience can also then help explain why killing a human being is worse than killing an insect. Both beings may be sentient but they are not equally sentient.

> [D]iffering degrees of sentience and mental sophistication make it reasonable to accord stronger moral status to some sentient beings than to others: for example, to protect vertebrate animals more carefully than insects, which appear to be only minimally sentient, and lacking in most of the more sophisticated mental capacities.
>
> (Warren 2000, p. 354)

Since the more sentient a being is, the more moral worth the being has, thus sentience can account both for moral differences between insects, animals, and human beings as well as the difference between early and late abortion or infanticide.

But differences in human sentience are not confined to the time of gestation. The kung fu master can put his arms around a burning cauldron, endure the searing of flesh, and carry the weighty object. The proverbial princess cannot stand the pea under her multiple mattresses. Many men cannot bear the least discomfort, and many women endure childbirth without anesthetic. Certain injuries and diseases greatly hinder the human capacity for pain, as do drugs of various kinds, as do differences in degrees of concentration and experience. Since adult human beings differ rather radically in their capacity for pain or pleasure, this should lead to the conclusion that they differ rather radically in terms of personhood. If degrees of sentience gives rise to degrees of rights, then not only are all human beings not equal, not all human persons are equal. Indeed, no two human persons have identical capacities for pain or pleasure. Our experiences of pains and pleasures are conditioned by our prior experiences, beliefs, and habits. Since no two human persons have the same experiences, beliefs, and habits, no two human persons have equal capacities for pleasure and pain, and therefore human persons do not have equal rights. This version of the sentience argument undermines equal rights for all persons.

Indeed, possessing sentience—at least sentience as understood as the capacity for pleasure and pain—does not seem necessary at all for having interests or rights. Imagine an alien or angel who was completely impervious to any physical pain. Although the angelic or alien constitution frees them from suffering, such beings could very well be more rationally perceptive than our best scientists (and perhaps equal even to our best philosophers!) and their communication skills might enable them to resolve stalemated world disputes. They would possess freedom and self-mastery that surpass the most virtuous human beings and display artistic talents to rival Raphael or Michelangelo. On the sentience account of interests and rights, these beings who surpass the achievements of humans in so many respects would have no interests or rights whatsoever. One retort would be that these beings, even if impervious to physical suffering, might experience emotional pain and on this basis they have interests and rights. Here a consideration of the Stoics might be in order. Their highest ideal was to make themselves immune from the tide of human emotion. Perhaps some succeeded in their goal or perhaps certain drugs or brain injuries could render someone physically and emotionally non-sentient. If this took place, would their interests or personhood really be in question?

Of course, we could use the term "sentience" in a different sense meaning not the ability to experience pleasure and pain, but rather the ability to have, for example, visual or audible sensations. The alien or angel in question would have these. But certainly sentience in either of these senses is not necessary for moral worth, for blind and deaf human beings are surely persons, albeit handicapped persons.

Imagine the case of an infant born in a condition of temporary unconsciousness. Since unconscious, the baby would lack sentience and thus also lack an interest in continuing life. Would it be permissible to terminate the baby's life? Bonnie Steinbock responds to this case,

> Because she is so close to being a normal baby, it is virtually impossible to treat her as anything else. In other words, although, strictly speaking, she does not have interests of her own, we treat her as if she did, because she is so close to having them.
>
> (1992, pp. 61–62)

But imagine the baby will gain consciousness in ten months. In this situation, a recently implanted human zygote is actually "closer," at least in time, to having sentience. Physiologically, the healthy newborn and the temporarily unconscious newborn are more similar to each than they are to the human zygote, but the sentience account excludes the importance of such physiological differences in favor of psychological differences.

In considering whether human beings who do not feel pain should be accorded the rights of persons, we are actually not dealing with merely imaginary examples. Although there have been very few human beings, most of them children, ever diagnosed with the condition, Congenital Insensitivity to Pain (CIPA) renders human beings totally insensitive to pain, for they lack proper beta-endorphins which modulate pain sensations.

Though this condition is very rare, it would be absurd to claim that because human beings suffering from this disease are unworthy of a life of dignity and respect, even if they were also deaf and blind and insensitive to pleasure as well. In sum, sentience is a poor marker of personhood because it could exclude beings that are obviously persons (such as temporarily unconscious newborns), it includes beings that are obviously not persons (such as insects) and could not secure the fundamental equality of persons even among adult, rationally functioning human beings, since such human beings differ rather radically in terms of sensitivity to pleasure and pain.

4.1.5 Human Appearance

The appearance of the human fetus could be seen as closely linked to human personhood as well. Early human fetuses (and embryos) don't have mouths, noses, eyes, or arms. They bear not the slightest resemblance to you or me. As Roger Wertheimer points out, "It is an amorphous speck of apparently coagulated protoplasm. It has no eyes or ears, no head at all. It can't walk or talk; you can't dress it or wash it. Why, it doesn't even qualify as a Barbie doll" (1971, p. 74). The spontaneous recognition that human beings can have for one another has been fundamental in determining their behavior. The appeal of appearance as a criterion for personhood may also be conveyed by the ethical work of Emmanuel Levinas in *Totality and Infinity* (1980) who points to the primacy of the face-to-face encounter with other humans in coming to moral awareness. Before the human fetus has a recognizable human form, it should be treated with the dignity corresponding to its appearance: merely as a protoplasmic blob at the beginning, perhaps as an animal of some type later in pregnancy, and finally as a human person when, and only when, it looks like a human person (English 1975, p. 241). When the human fetus's appearance is suitably human looking would again be a matter of some dispute. Perhaps this occurs in the first trimester or perhaps only near the end of pregnancy. But whatever one's answer to this question, on this view the human fetus becomes a human person if and only if it has human appearance.

How might someone opposed to abortion respond? It certainly cannot be denied that no embryo or very early fetus will ever star in a Gerber commercial. In terms of looks and the ability to stir unreflective human emotion, a zygote, embryo, or early fetus utterly fails. However, such feelings are far from morally decisive. As Roger Wertheimer notes slaveholders simply could not believe that African Americans:

> were full-fledged human beings, the sort of creatures that it is wrong to kill or enslave was a claim he found incredible. He would be inclined to, and actually did, simply point to Negroes and say: "Look at them! Can't you see the difference between them and us?" And the fact is that at one time that argument had an undeniable

power as undeniable as the perceptual differences it appealed to. Check your own perceptions. Ask yourself whether you really, in a purely phenomenological sense, see a member of another race in the same way you see a member of your own. . . . The parallels with the abortion controversy are palpable.

(1971, p. 84)

Looks can be deceiving, and obviously bear no decisive or necessary relationship to personhood. A burn victim whose charred appearance renders him revolting or even not recognizably human, nevertheless still has as much a right to life as any supermodel. The woman whose face is destroyed by cancer or the man missing limbs and facial skin due to leprosy has as much a right not to be killed as the prom queen or *People* magazine's "sexiest man alive." The look of human form is not important in determining who is a person, since there are or very well may be non-human persons. We should base ethical judgments, indeed judgments in general, not on what appears to be the case, but on what is in reality the case.

4.1.6 Brain Development

According to Baruch Brody, one cannot be a member of *Homo sapiens* without a brain, and so if a functioning brain is not present then no human being is present, and therefore no human person (1975). So until the development of a brain, about six weeks after conception within the first trimester, the human fetus would lack rights but after this point the being in utero would be a human being and also a person. Early methods of abortion such as RU-486 would be permissible on this view, but methods of later abortion, including all surgical abortions after eight weeks, would be impermissible. Why is the brain the essential characteristic of a human person? Well just as, on some views, brain death defines the end of a human person, so too would brain life, an existing functioning brain, mark the beginning of a human person. As Boonin notes in explaining this argument, just as removing one of three sides from a figure makes the figure no longer a triangle, so too adding a side to a two-sided figure makes it a triangle. Similarly as human persons we die when the brain dies; so too we live when the brain begins to live (Savulescu 2002). Without a functioning brain, a being is either not yet a human person (an early fetus) or no longer a human person (a lifeless corpse).

Should the emergence of the brain indicate the beginning of a human person just as brain death signals the end of the human person? Perhaps the most powerful objection to this argument rests on the rejection of whole brain death as an adequate criterion of the death of a human being (Miller and Truog 2009; Shewmon 1998, 2001, 2004, 2009). A principal reason given for supposing that whole brain death is the death of a human being is that all vital organs of brain dead human beings imminently and inexorably begin to shut down, despite the most aggressive medical treatment. This empirical claim has been undermined to a large extent by contrary empirical evidence. Speaking of whole brain death (not simply "higher-brain death"), neurologist D. Alan Shewmon argues:

> The mainstream rationale for equating brain death (BD) with death is that the brain confers integrative unity upon the body, transforming it from a mere collection of organs and tissues to an organism as a whole. In support of this conclusion, the impressive list of the brain's myriad integrative functions is often cited. Upon closer examination, and after operational definition of terms, however, one discovers that most integrative functions of the brain are actually not somatically integrating, and, conversely, most integrative functions of the body are not brain-mediated. With respect to organism-level vitality, the brain's role is more modulatory than constitutive, enhancing the quality and survival potential of a presupposedly living organism. Integrative unity of a complex organism is an inherently nonlocalizable, holistic feature involving the mutual interaction among all the parts, not a top-down coordination imposed by one part upon a passive multiplicity of other parts. Loss of somatic integrative unity is not a physiologically tenable rationale for equating BD with death of the organism as a whole.
>
> (2001, p. 457)

Shewmon also cites a case in which he had personal clinical experience. He examined a boy whom he calls "TK" who became "brain dead" at age 4 and was still alive, at home, at age 19 (Shewmon 1999, p. 323). The example of TK would seem to indicate that brain death is not the death of a human being, nor does it imminently lead to the death of a human organism.

Even if brain death is a legitimate way to determine death, it may not be a good way to determine when life or personhood begins. Stephen Schwarz points out that brain death is used as a criterion to determine death precisely because after brain death a human being no longer will function as a person in the future. This lack of potentiality leads to the determination of death. On the other hand, if there is potentiality for normal human activity, the case looks much different. If the brain is only temporarily not functioning properly, and the human being will be able to flourish in the future, then brain death has not taken place. But this is precisely the case with the typical human fetus or embryo whose lack of function is not permanent but only temporary due to a lack of maturity. So fetal status is akin to being in a temporary coma from which someone will entirely recover, rather than being brain dead (Schwarz 1990).

One might also ask: why is the brain of such tremendous importance for personhood? Earthworms, wasps, and ants have brains, but they hardly count as persons. The alien or angel problem arises once again. If they arrived on the scene, doing their marvelous works, but lacked a brain, would it really make sense to deny that they have personhood? These angels or aliens would obviously be persons, even though lacking a brain: so having a brain is not essential to being a person.

In addition, if one holds that having a brain at all marks the beginning of personhood, then it begins well within the first trimester. On the other hand, if a full completed brain is required, then personhood would begin much too late. Indeed, brain development hardly stops at birth, but continues well into childhood. Understood in its broadest sense, brain development, or learning, can continue one's entire life. As Singer writes, marking the beginning of human life in terms of brain development is a:

> convenient fiction that turns an evidently living being into one that legally is not alive. Instead of accepting such fictions, we should recognize that the fact that a being is human, and alive, does not in itself tell us whether it is wrong to take that being's life.
>
> (Singer 1994, p. 105)

Thus, from a biological standpoint, the brain has no essential connection with the beginning of a human being; from a moral standpoint, the brain has no essential connection with personhood. Other people hold that the brain is essential for persistent human identity as an individual over time, but not necessarily for personhood. This important perspective will be treated in chapter five.

4.1.7 Implantation

The importance of implantation, when the embryo embeds in the uterine wall, is linked to the issue of abortion (particularly very early chemical abortion), the fate of human embryos created through *in vitro* fertilization not implanted in the womb ("spare" human embryos), and to therapeutic cloning, so just a word about cloning is in order. A distinction is sometimes drawn between therapeutic cloning and reproductive cloning. Therapeutic cloning creates a new human embryo, with the same genome as the "parent" who is cloned, but destroys this human embryo in research before it is implanted in a woman's uterus. Reproductive cloning creates a human embryo for the sake of implanting the embryo in a maternal womb to be born. So if human personhood begins at implantation, and not before, then therapeutic cloning would be permissible, even though it destroys a human embryo. U.S. Senator Orrin Hatch expresses this view in its most popular form when he says that a human life worthy of respect begins "in a woman's womb, not a Petri dish."

But slogans are not arguments. So why then is implantation important? Bernard Nathanson in his book *Aborting America* defends this conclusion in the following way. Before earlier detection of pregnancy was possible, common law outlawed abortion when pregnancy was known to exist and this point, as we have seen, came at quickening. With the progress of science, we can now determine the existence of a pregnancy well before quickening. However, the earliest way to detect pregnancy now available will only detect pregnancy following implantation, at which time a woman's body releases a hormone (HCG) which allows a pregnancy to be detected. As Nathanson notes:

> Biochemically, this is when alpha [the human zygote] announces its presence as part of the human community by means of its hormonal messages, which we now have the technology to receive. We also know biochemically that it is an independent organism distinct from the mother.
>
> (1979, p. 216)

The arrival of the embryo in utero was known in centuries past only through quickening but can now be determined through pregnancy tests which can detect a pregnancy only following implantation. The "implantation" criterion would seem to allow for abortion only in the earliest stage of pregnancy; yet it would also seem thereby to legitimate de facto abortions by means of the birth control pill, which can work by inhibiting implantation of a human zygote, as well as the use of some "emergency" contraceptives which also prevent implantation.

Does implantation in the uterus mark the moment when mere humanity ends and personhood begins, since only at implantation is the embryo detectable by current technology? Choice of implantation as a marker of personhood is ironic because usually it is argued that being connected to the mother makes the human being in utero a non-person, but in this case not being connected to the mother makes the embryo a non-person. In any case, implantation has no essential connection to personhood. If artificial wombs become a reality, it would be possible for a human being to develop from conception to infancy without being connected to a mother. Would it follow that such children never attain personhood? We can also imagine alien or angelic persons never implanted in a womb.

However, a closer examination of Nathanson's argument is in order. (For the record, Nathason later came to believe that personhood began at conception (2001)). The importance of "recognition" could be understood in two very different ways. It could either mean that this particular human embryo actually is recognized, or that this particular human embryo could, in principle, be recognized by someone outside the womb even if not actually recognized by anyone. At least from Nathanson's account of recognition, the first alternative certainly won't do, since it has happened that women go into labor still not knowing they are pregnant, or even give birth in utter amazement that a child has emerged from them. Nathanson doesn't want to hold that all these women who get pregnancy tests and know they are pregnant are carrying human persons but women who don't know they are pregnant are not carrying human persons. A difference in the knowledge of these women or their physicians makes no difference whatsoever to what the human fetus is or whether the human fetus is a person. So the first possibility is excluded. The second possibility, that personhood arises whenever any given human embryos can be detected, pushes personhood before implantation since at least some human embryos can be detected before implantation.

Another strategy for arguing that implantation has importance is simply to note that an implanted embryo is closer to realizing its potential than a non-implanted zygote, and so there is a morally significant difference between abortion post-implantation on the one hand and abortifacient or embryo experimentation on the other hand. The implanted embryo is closer to realizing its personhood, and so merits a greater respect (Coleman 2004, p. 110).

The plausibility of this argument trades on an ambiguity. In terms of physical development, an implanted embryo is closer to realizing its potential to become a mature human being, just as a 1-year-old is closer than a newborn. But it is not obvious that being closer to maturity makes any moral difference whatsoever in terms of the right to life. On the other hand, in terms of moral personhood, precisely at issue is whether an unimplanted embryo has the same right to life as an implanted embryo, or a human fetus, or a newborn, or a 1-year-old. To argue that the implanted embryo is "closer to realizing its potential," in this sense, is simply to beg the question at issue.

An additional problem with implantation includes over-inclusivity, for if implantation in a uterus alone makes a being into a person than personhood must be extended to all those animals, such as rats, that develop their young in utero.

Of course, one may very well say that although rat embryos implant in a uterus, this fact is not significant since it is a rat embryo and not a human embryo. But of course, this is to attribute moral significance, nearly decisive moral significance, to being a member of the species *Homo sapiens*—and to concede exactly what is typically denied by the conventional pro-choice view.

4.2 The Developmental View

A pro-choice response to the critiques given thus far of various possible candidates for marking the transition to personhood might take the form of the *gradualist* view, also sometimes known as the *pluralistic* view, the *developmental* view, or the *multi-criterial* approach as advocated by Warren's later work on abortion (1997). Although each of the proposed criteria might fail as sufficient conditions for personhood taken individually, taken together they lead to the conclusion that the right to life gradually increases in strength as the pregnancy continues. Indeed, rather than pitting viability against quickening, the ability to move spontaneously against sentience, and recognizable human form against formation of the brain and so forth, in the gradualist view all these views could be combined. The more similar a being is in these respects to full-fledged persons like ourselves, the greater the protection it is due (Green 2001, p. 62). Each of these marks has been criticized as weak in part because each either includes too many beings as persons (e.g., cockroaches are sentient, mosquitoes have brains) or excludes too many beings as persons (prematurely born infants don't have conscious experiences, paralyzed adults cannot move). However, even if any given argument in favor of personhood arising in the womb might be over- or under-inclusive and so not a sufficient condition for personhood taken individually, the gradualist view builds upon each argument in turn combining the various arguments.

One might compare the gradualist argument to the construction of a rope. Just as a single thread is easily broken, so too the human embryo of only a few cells has almost no moral worth and can be destroyed without ethical qualm. When more threads are bound with the original one, a string begins to exist that is more difficult to break than any thread taken individually but nevertheless may be fairly easily broken. So too, abortion early in pregnancy is more serious than mere embryo destruction but is still easily justified. When still more threads are added a string becomes a rope which is difficult to split, similarly, an abortion late in pregnancy would only be justified in rather extreme circumstances. Each of the stages of development from conception through birth are like threads added which gradually make the claims of the human fetus stronger and stronger until shortly before birth the human being in utero has a right to life equal to that of any other person. Although each individual thread of argument may be weak considered in itself, either by being under-inclusive (e.g., by not including infants or handicapped adult humans) or over-inclusive (e.g., by including worms or cockroaches), when taken together these threads point to the increasing moral importance of the human fetus over time.

Indeed, the rights of the human fetus should grow along with age and development, just as do other rights of humans after birth. We have many examples of the gradual attainment of rights. Indeed, in the United States at fifteen and a half, people gain the right to drive a car with a learner's permit and its restrictions. At sixteen, a human being is said to be sufficiently mature to have the right to drive a car alone. At eighteen, the right to vote is gained and for men the possibility of being drafted for military service. At twenty-one, at least in most states, a person attains the right legally to drink alcohol. At twenty-five, a U.S. citizen may serve in the U.S. House of Representatives, at thirty in the U.S. Senate, and at thirty-five as President of the United States. So too with the human being between conception and birth, we have a gradual attainment of rights which become greater as age and physical development increase. A human being just following conception has little or no rights but a human being just before birth has greater rights. The right to life then is a right, unlike voting, that one attains sometime between conception and birth. The gradualist approach holds that the newly conceived embryo has no moral value (or extremely little) but this value increases throughout the course of pregnancy and fetal development. The way of accounting for the value of the fetus is pluralistic in that it takes into account a plurality of considerations rather than assuming that one simple characteristic grants the human fetus personhood. Thus, the gradualist view steers between the extremes of claiming personhood begins at conception and claiming personhood begins at birth by finding a virtuous mean—personhood gradually arises between conception and birth. This view also explains why early abortions are less problematic than late-term abortions, partial-birth abortions, or infanticide. The later in gestation, the greater the moral value possessed by the human fetus.

4.3 A Critique of the Developmental View

How in turn might this gradualist, pluralistic, or developmental view be criticized? Although the gradualist view is a mean between the extremes of holding personhood begins at conception and personhood begins at birth, Aristotle pointed out in book two of the *Nicomachean Ethics* that not everything admits of a virtuous mean. The mathematical mean between killing 100 innocent people and killing no innocent people would be killing 50 innocent people—but this mean is not virtuous but vicious.

One can easily accept, however, that it is just and right that some rights are gradually attained with age and maturity without holding that all rights are attained with age and maturity. Although ultimately affirming the permissibility of abortion, Roger Wertheimer is skeptical about comparing the right to life to other rights attained later in human development (1971, p. 83). The radical difference between the right to life and other rights, such as the right to vote, does not rest merely on the fact that without life one cannot exercise any other right whatsoever. Voting, driving, and serving as an elected official are examples of rights that have corresponding responsibilities. Five-year-olds cannot have a right to drive or to vote or to serve in office because they cannot discharge the responsibilities that come along with these rights. On the contrary, the right to life does not implicitly contain any corresponding responsibilities—and so may be enjoyed by those who cannot discharge any duties—like children before the age of reason or mentally handicapped adults. So although it makes sense that some rights are gradually attained with maturity, since these rights have corresponding responsibilities, it does not follow that all rights are of this kind.

Even if we could distinguish various kinds of rights, perhaps the rope analogy makes sense. As illustrated by this analogy, should we link human development in the womb with an increasingly significant moral status for the human fetus? One problem with this view is that human development hardly ends with birth. The gradualist position should lead us to hold that killing a 20-year-old requires a greater justification than killing a 14-year-old and that killing a 14-year-old requires a greater justification than killing a 6-year-old, and so on. If moral status is linked to physiological development and decline, killing a 50-year-old would require less justification than killing a 30-year-old. But of course this is nonsense. All human persons have equal rights to life, and all murders as such are equally wrong. Human development and moral status are simply not linked in the manner proposed by the gradualist position.

A second weakness of the rope analogy for the gradualist view is the comparison of the various arguments in favor of personhood to threads which though weak taken individually make an increasingly strong case. For unlike a thread, an argument that is invalid or unsound does not have any "strength" which could then be added to other arguments the sum of which would amount to a stronger case for one's view. If for instance Tooley is correct that viability, spontaneous movement, and human form do not distinguish mere human beings from persons, then putting viability, spontaneous movement, and human form together would not make the gradualist case any stronger.

Let's say I revive a formerly widespread prejudice and argue human beings from Ireland are not fully persons. My reasoning? The Irish are not fully persons because (1) they have red hair, (2) they are Roman Catholic, and (3) they are economically disadvantaged. You point out to me scores of blond, Protestant, and rich Irishmen and note further that these three characteristics have absolutely no relationship to personhood. My case for the Irish lacking personhood is not strengthened in the least by calling your attention to the fact that I have three (or three hundred) such arguments that when taken together constitute an increasingly stronger case for my view. An invalid or unsound argument counts for nothing. Such an argument is a philosophical zero, and even an infinite number of zeros never adds up to more than zero. A thread has some strength; a bad argument has none. There is no reason to think that individually unsound arguments against personhood somehow when taken as a group demonstrate that not all human beings should be respected as persons, whether those human beings are living in Ireland or living in utero.

One reason some people hold the developmental view is that they believe later abortion is worse than early abortion, and this seems to be explained by linking the physiological development of the human being in utero with the moral worth. The more physically developed the human fetus, the more valuable the fetus is, and the worse abortion becomes (Warnock 2004, pp. 79–80).

In his article "Late- vs. Early Term Abortion," Andrew Peach notes that other things being equal we need not appeal to the developmental view in order to recognize five important moral differences between late abortion and early abortion (Peach 2007). First, just as murder by torturous means is worse than murder by painless means because of the additional evil of inflicting grievous suffering, so too late-term abortion involving fetal pain (e.g., partial-birth abortion) is worse than killing of the unborn that does not cause pain (e.g., lethal embryonic research). Of course, it is possible to remove this difference by simply anesthetizing the human fetus prior to the late-term abortion procedure, but in second or third trimester abortions as typically performed this difference remains. Others might object that even the early fetus experiences pain, but the typical advocate of abortion denies this, so Peach's argument would work at least dialectically on his opponent's supposition. In any case, it is certainly true that *some* killing of early human life (say, killing embryos for research purposes) would involve no fetal or embryonic pain and therefore would be distinguishable from other forms of killing (partial-birth abortion) that as typically performed involve pain on a normal human fetus.

Second, Peach points out that the more easily an obligation can be met the worse it is not to meet it. To fail to save a man's life by refusing to run two blocks is worse than to fail to save his life by refusing to run ten miles. But to finish carrying a pregnancy already several months along is easier *ceteris paribus* than to carry a pregnancy the entire nine months, thus later abortion is worse than early abortion.

However, as a counter-example, consider a woman suddenly having to endure bed rest for the last three months of pregnancy or undergoing health problems in later pregnancy who might very well experience the pregnancy as more difficult and requiring greater effort than a healthy woman going through an entire pregnancy. Nevertheless, Peach's general point would still hold if it is understood as defending a *prima facie* moral difference between early term abortion and late-term abortion.

Third, he argues that in early abortion the identity of the human fetus is more easily misunderstood while later in pregnancy the humanity of the unborn is more evident. There is some initial plausibility (though upon investigation it is not true) that the human embryo is just a "bunch of cells." However, fetal movement (sometimes hiccups), vivid 3D ultrasound and sonograms of later pregnancy make the humanity of the unborn harder to deny. Thus, it is more difficult to appeal to inculpable ignorance when aborting later in pregnancy.

Again, there may be cases when this difference is not in play. Someone well versed in the facts of fetal development may be more culpable for having an early abortion than a mentally handicapped woman aborting later in pregnancy. Still, if the point is to make a *prima facie* case that there is greater culpability for later abortion than for early abortion, the point remains true despite differences in cases where other things are not equal.

Fourth, early in pregnancy, the shock and panic aroused by the initial news lessens the culpability of those who choose abortion in this state. However, as time goes on, passions cool and therefore late term abortion becomes *ceteris paribus* more deliberate and therefore worse. Finally, as the pregnancy continues, presumably the attachment between mother and child grows making any "detachment" all the more traumatic and morally problematic. To end a marriage after four weeks differs from ending it after four decades. One need not deny the equal rights of all innocent human beings whatever their stage of development in order to account for the intuition that later abortion is typically worse in some respects than early abortion.

One difficulty with this argument is that it does not apply in all cases to distinguish early from later abortion. In some cases of late-term abortion, the mother may wish to terminate the pregnancy because of a diagnosis of fetal handicap only found later in pregnancy. The emotional trauma brought on by the news of a malformed, unborn child late in pregnancy may be no less severe than the distress brought about by an unwanted pregnancy discovered early. In addition, it can happen that a woman with irregular cycles or obesity only discovers that she is pregnant in the second or third trimester. Still, these exceptions do not undermine the general thesis that late-term abortion is more morally problematic than early term abortion *ceteris paribus*.

Fifth and finally, Peach points to the fact that, in general, late-term miscarriages are experienced as more traumatic than early miscarriages.

> Even if they feel or have judged that abortion is a necessary evil, all things considered, their sense of remorse and loss would have to be more palpable or intense given the level of development of the child; what has been taken away cannot plausibly be denied. This must be particularly true for the woman, whose attachment to the person in her womb presumably develops as the child develops. Just as, in general, late-term miscarriages are likely to impact a woman (or couple) more severely than early term ones, late-term abortions must surely impact a woman (or couple) more severely than early term ones.
>
> (2007, p. 138)

Generally, it does seem to be the case that late miscarriages are more traumatic for women (and couples) than early miscarriage. Does it follow that late abortions are morally worse than early abortions? Does an attachment develop between the mother and the child through the course of pregnancy such that the greater the attachment, the worse it is to detach? Generally, the length of a relationship seems to have some bearing on the loss involved when the relationship ends. To end a marriage after three weeks involves a less serious loss than ending it after three decades. Though Peach's five arguments do not show that later abortion is *always* worse than early abortion in terms of circumstances and moral culpability—though they are equally unjust in terms of being the intentional killing of an innocent unborn human person—it would seem that Peach's arguments are sound so long as they are understood as *ceteris paribus* considerations. If the arguments are sound, we can explain why later abortion is generally viewed as worse than early abortion without denying the equal basic value of innocent human beings in whatever stage of development.

Another argument against fetal personhood and in favor of the developmental view is that people generally do distinguish between the killing of a fetus, the killing of a newborn, and the killing of an adult. "If viable fetuses come within the scope of the constraint against harmful using, it should be as seriously wrong, other things being equal, to kill a viable fetus as it is to kill an older child or adult" (McMahan 2007, pp. 18–19).

On a pro-life view, there is a certain equality in all cases of intentionally killing innocent human beings at any age of their development, embryonic, fetal, neo-natal, adolescent, or adult. All such killing violates the right to life, which is equal for all innocent human persons. It does not follow from this that killing an embryo and killing an adult are equally wrong in all other respects. Often an action will be wrong for more than one reason, and killing an older child or innocent adult is wrong not only because it is intentional killing of the innocent but also because, characteristically, such killing unreasonably thwarts the individual's life-plans and induces fear as well as personal loss in those who cared for the deceased. Similarly, killing a regular person and killing the President of the United States are equally wrong as killing. The regular person and the President have equal rights to live. However, unlike killing a regular person, killing the President may also generate global instability, upset millions of people, and perhaps even prompt massive retaliation or world war. These factors make the assassination of any world leader more grievously wrong than killing a private citizen, but, nevertheless, killing the President and killing a private citizen are equally wrong with respect to the violation of the right to life. Analogously, there is no need to appeal to the developmental view, to differences in fundamental moral status, to explain why it is worse to kill a human adult than to kill a human fetus. Unlike killing a human fetus, killing an adult normally involves the additional evils of unreasonably thwarting the person's life plans, inducing fear in others, and depriving others of the deceased person's company and contributions.

Having examined the pros and cons of the most important arguments that personhood arises during gestation, let us turn now to the next logical possibility. If personhood does not arise after birth, or at birth, or between birth and conception, then the next possibility would be that personhood arises at conception. Does the completion of fertilization bring about a new human person? The next chapter focuses on this difficult question and with it the centrality of human personal identity.

5   Does Personhood Begin at Conception?

In order to answer any question, it helps to get clarity about what exactly is being asked. Indeed, this chapter addresses not one but two questions: Is every human being a person? And, do human beings begin to exist at conception? The first is a moral question that inquires as to who is a member of the moral community; the second is a biological question that seeks to know when human life begins.

In asking whether every human being is a person, we should make clear that this is not simply a question about abortion. The question of which human beings we ought to treat with respect also comes into play in ethical questions too numerous to list exhaustively: questions about race relations, national rivalries, religious conflicts, slavery, criminal punishment, conjoined twins, deformed human beings, handicapped human beings, and ethnic cleansing, to mention a few.

5.1 Are All Human Beings Persons?

Almost everyone agrees that some human beings are persons, including anyone reading this book. If there is no ethically relevant difference between you and another human being, then it is unfair that you should be treated as a person but not the other human being. If the basic argument of previous chapters has been successful, then attempts to distinguish human persons from mere human beings have failed. There is no ethically relevant difference between human beings of various stages of development that renders some human beings non-persons. If the dignity and value of the human person does not begin after birth, nor at birth, nor sometime during gestation, then human personhood begins at conception. Thus, all human beings are also human persons.

Some people object to the view that all human beings are persons in the following way. "Assertion of the superiority of our own kind, whether defined by species membership, race, gender, nationality, or religion, seems not only unjustified, but unjustifiable" (Harris & Holm 2003, p. 119). Jukka Varelius raises the objection that human dignity is inherently unjust towards other species. "Furthermore, it could be maintained that granting all and only members of the human species special dignity is speciesism and, accordingly, morally on a par with such isms as sexism and racism" (Varelius 2009, p. 38). We should therefore reject granting dignity, and the rights that go with that dignity, to all human beings as inherently unfair to non-humans.

This often-used objection against human dignity, equal basic rights for all human beings, rests on two confusions. The first is merely linguistic. From the truth that racism and sexism are wrong, we cannot simply add "ism" to some class of characteristics to create a morally illegitimate point of demarcation. After all, advocates for abortion rights themselves characteristically endorse either sentientism (valuing sentient beings over non-sentient beings) or autonomism (valuing autonomous beings over non-autonomous beings). To simply assert that denying dignity on the basis of species is as morally dubious as denying dignity on the basis of race or sex is to beg the question—which is precisely whether non-human animals are equal in dignity to human beings.

Second, even if speciesism is ethically problematic, a commitment to the dignity of all human beings does not involve a denial of dignity to any other class of non-human beings simply because they are not human. Defenders of the dignity of all human beings need not believe, and characteristically do not believe, that *only* humans have dignity. Many critics of abortion believe, for example, that God the Father, the Son, and the Holy Spirit as well as angels are persons with dignity. Even aside from religious beliefs, it is possible that there are many other beings in the universe, such as intelligent aliens, that have dignity, for there very well may be many other beings in the universe who have a rational nature, and therefore have dignity even if they are non-human. Of course, such beings would not have human dignity, since they are not human, but they would have dignity and rights. The belief that *all* human beings have dignity simply does not imply a commitment to the view that *only* human beings have dignity. Being human is a sufficient but not a necessary condition for having rights. In other words, the question of animal rights is simply not answered by a commitment to the equal, intrinsic dignity of all human beings.

Although often linked with discussions of the rights of non-human beings, holding that "every human being is a person" (EHP) does not imply *anything* about the moral status of those that are not human. One could believe EHP and that *only* human beings are persons. One could accept EHP and also hold that animals have moral status and should be treated well for their own sake even though they lack *equal* moral status with human beings. One could hold that EHP and also hold that some (or all) animals should also be treated as equal persons to humans or that alien beings might exist and are also equal persons. One could even believe that all forms of life in the universe (including plants and insects) are equally sacred and should all be treated as persons. EHP is compatible with holding that the human beings have the *greatest* moral worth in comparison to all other living beings, *equal* moral worth in comparison to other living beings, or the *least* moral worth in comparison to other persons. So, one can answer the question "Is every human being a person?" affirmatively without taking any stand whatsoever on animal rights or alien rights. To link these questions unnecessarily is to make a difficult question much more difficult.

5.1.1 Personhood as Endowment or Performance?

The moral question "Is every human being a person?" is an extremely important one considered in itself and not just because it appears in so many ethical controversies. Indeed, in answering this question, one presupposes or reinforces at least implicitly a general theory of personhood. Drawing upon the work of the philosopher Robert Spitzer in his book *Healing the Culture* (2000) and John Kavanaugh in *Who Count as Persons?* (2001), we can contrast the *endowment account* of personhood with the *performance account* of personhood. The endowment account holds that each human being has inherent, moral worth simply by virtue of the kind of being it is. By endowment, I mean that the being in question has an intrinsic, dynamic orientation towards self-expressive activity (Clarke 1995, p. 105). Beings with endowments that orient them towards moral values, such as rationality, autonomy, and respect, thereby merit inclusion as members of the moral community. The performance account, including the various versions examined in previous chapters, denies this and holds that a being is to be accorded respect, if and only if, the being functions in a given way. There are numerous and conflicting accounts of what this function is, but some of the proposed candidates include: self-awareness, rationality, sentience, desirability, ethnicity, economic productivity, gender, nationality, native language, beauty, age, health, religion, race, ethnicity, fertility, birth, and national origin.

With respect to human beings, the endowment view is *inclusive*; the performance view is *exclusive*. According to the inclusive view, all human beings regardless of any consideration whatsoever have fundamental dignity and are therefore owed respect. According to the exclusive view, not all human beings deserve respect and share fundamental dignity, but rather only those human beings possessing particular characteristics. The exclusive view does not specify how many characteristics generate personhood. Some think a single characteristic grants personhood while others claim a multiplicity. Indeed, there is little agreement on which characteristics comprehensively constitute personhood. Those who advocate self-awareness, rationality, or sentience may dispute with those who advocate desirability, economic productivity, or ability to communicate, and they, in turn, will also disagree with those who believe nationality, native language, or self-motivated activity confer personhood. All these would disagree with those who advocate beauty, age, health, religion, race, fertility, or birth as that which confers personhood. So the performance view is not exclusive in the sense that it requires that any particular function confers personhood, rather it is exclusive in the sense that it sets a requirement of performance as the test of personhood.

Note that these performance tests are characteristically *qualitative* measurements by which human beings can and do differ by degree. Human beings are more or less intelligent, more or less sentient, more or less physically developed, more or less independent, more or less self-aware, and more or less wanted by others. Obviously, such views exclude some human beings from personhood. However, not only does the performance view deny that all human beings are created equal and endowed with certain inalienable rights, but the view implies that not all persons are fundamentally equal. How could we possibly arrive at the conclusion that *all persons* are equal if not all persons equally possess the attribute that leads to personhood? If what gives a person dignity and value is quality X, and quality X comes in various degrees, then there should be degrees of dignity and value among persons. The more I have of X, the greater dignity I have *as a person*. Alan Gewirth calls this the Principle of Proportionality (Gewirth 1978, p. 121). Thus, not only does the performance view divide human beings against one another, performance valuation even *divides persons among themselves*. For example, if sentience gives rise to rights, and not all human persons are equally sentient, then not all human persons enjoy equal rights. If the performance account is accepted, it is unclear how one could ever affirm that all human persons are equal before the law or morally equal other than by an arbitrary fiat that can be just as arbitrarily rescinded.

An advocate for the sentience view could hold that even though sentience does come in degrees, one is either sentient or one is not. Similarly, people have better and worse vision, but one is either totally blind or one is not. So, if a being has sentience, even if it is to a very small degree, then the being has moral worth, indeed equal moral worth with every other sentient being.

A difficulty with this view is that wasps, ants, locusts, and mosquitos also are sentient beings. So, if all sentient beings have moral worth, then these insects have moral worth, indeed, equal moral worth to human beings. This is obviously absurd. No one thinks that insects should have equal rights to human persons.

Some defenders of abortion recognize the problem. Pushed by questions posed by Tim Mulgan, McMahan expresses skepticism about the possibility of basing the *equal* moral worth of human persons on properties that are *unequal* among human persons, such as psychological capacities or ethical achievement. He notes, as mentioned previously,

All this leaves me profoundly uncomfortable. It seems virtually unthinkable to abandon our egalitarian commitments, or even to accept that they might be justified only in some indirect way—for example, because it is for the best, all things considered, to treat all people as equals and to inculcate the belief that all are indeed one another's moral equals, even though in reality they are not. Yet the challenges to the equal wrongness thesis, which is a central element of liberal egalitarian morality, support Mulgan's skepticism about the compatibility of our all-or-nothing egalitarian beliefs with the fact that the properties on which our moral status appears to supervene are all matters of degree. It is hard to avoid the sense that our egalitarian commitments rest on distressingly insecure foundations.

(2008, p. 104)

McMahan himself acknowledges how recklessly discriminatory it would be, both politically and socially, to push to deny the fundamental equality of a group of human persons. The logical implications of performance accounts of personhood undermine not only the rights of a certain class of human beings but undermine the basic equality of all human persons.

By contrast, the endowment account applies equally to all human beings who, despite their manifest differences in rational function, for example, remain oriented towards reason and freedom, even when this orientation cannot be expressed because of immaturity, illness, sleep, or disability. To be oriented toward reason and freedom is to have one's flourishing and welfare consists in enjoying certain kinds of goods (e.g, friendship, knowing the truth) that can only be achieved through the exercise of reason and freedom. The flourishing of human beings consists in lives constituted by reason and freedom, even if in certain cases this flourishing is impeded by unfortunate circumstances, such as disease, or by the deliberate choice of others, such as radical lobotomy. Unfortunately, many human beings do not yet share in human flourishing.

Indeed, it is impossible to find *two* human beings, let alone an entire nation of human beings, who are equal in regard to strength, intelligence, beauty, virtue, and other valuable characteristics. Even a single one of these characteristics, rational functioning, is not shared equally by any two human beings, for emotional intelligence, prudential reasoning, mathematical ability, aptitude for physics, philosophical acumen, and literary gifts all come in degrees. If human beings are in any way fundamentally equal, this equality must rest on something they share equally. The equality problem is solved.

If every human being is recognized as a person, based simply on personal endowment, then the "episodic problem," where the personhood of a being comes and goes, is also avoided. Finally, valuing personal endowment avoids the problem of various forms of under-inclusiveness and over-inclusiveness. If we understand a person as a member of a kind of being that is rational and free, and since each and every human being is a member of a kind of being (namely human beings) that is rational and free, then all these problems are avoided. One's biological humanity is not episodic, so we don't face the problem of one and the same human being getting personhood and then losing it and then regaining it again and so on. Personal performance accounts must in fact rely implicitly on some version of personal endowment for their plausibility. In addition, biological humanity is characteristically *equally shared* by all human beings, so if one's humanity grants personhood, then all human persons are *fundamentally equal* in a moral sense and should enjoy fundamental equal rights before the law. Basing the personhood of humans on their shared humanity is not over-inclusive, including beings like worms that are obviously not persons, nor under-inclusive, excluding human beings who are in comas, physically or mentally handicapped, sleeping, or under anesthesia.

Indeed, performance accounts of personhood characteristically must rely on corrupted versions of the endowment account. No one asserts that *actually* feeling pleasure or pain makes a being have interests; rather they assert that the *capacity* to feel pleasure and pain makes interests. No one asserts that only *while performing* the activity of reasoning is one a person, rather the *ability* to reason makes one a person. No one asserts that one must *currently desire* something to have a right to life; rather they assert that one must at least *dispositionally* desire something. Others appeal to some species-specific necessary condition for rational functioning (neural architecture), rejecting a species-independent condition necessary for rational performance, namely rational endowment. In other words, everyone at least tacitly admits that pure performance accounts are implausible and that endowment of some kind (ability, capacity, disposition) is not just necessary but sufficient for the right to life. Rational endowment is nothing other than the capacity, ability, or disposition (though perhaps not realizable) enjoyed only by whole, living beings whose active self-development is aimed towards and whose flourishing consists in freedom and rationality.

Nor should an endowment account of personhood be seen as some sectarian religious view. Endowment accounts are already implicitly at work in the medical arts via the very concept of pathology. Pathology is not a simply lack of something. Rather, a pathology is an incapacity, inability, or failure to realize a disposition which, in the relevant circumstances, can and ought to be realized given the endowment of the being in question. Birds that do not speak are not thereby suffering a pathology. A human being of six years old who cannot speak following an accident *is* suffering a pathology, physical or mental. The practice of medicine, both for humans and non-humans, can and does appeal to endowments, what a being can and should be able to do given the requisite conditions, maturity, and support.

How does flourishing relate to our moral duties? Aside from just punishments, it is a violation of your rights when someone intentionally undermines your flourishing or what is necessary for your flourishing. To kill you is to undermine your flourishing because being alive is necessary for you to flourish and is itself partially constitutive of your flourishing, so it is wrong to kill you. This is true not simply of you as an individual but of all others whose flourishing is similar to yours. So, it is wrong to kill any other being who shares flourishing-like-yours. This norm then would exclude the intentional killing of all innocent human beings and any other being sharing flourishing-like-yours.

S. Matthew Liao offers a distinct, but compatible answer to the question of whether all human beings are persons. According to this view, personhood is tied to moral agency—not that all persons are always acting as moral agents or could at every moment act as moral agents, but that all persons actually have the genetic basis to be moral agents. Liao suggests that all human beings have rights in virtue of having the genetic basis for moral agency (2010a, p. 168). The genetic basis for moral agency is species neutral, in so far as other non-human animals may or may not have the genetic basis for moral agency. It is an actual, identifiable, physical attribute of the individual. The genetic basis of moral agency is not a matter of potentiality, but rather of what a being actually possesses. This basis is not just being a member of a group some of whose members have this attribute, but a case of the individual himself or herself having the attribute. Furthermore,

> since the genetic basis for moral agency is only a sufficient condition for rightholding, it avoids the intuitive cost of denying the status of rightholding to those non-human animals or other beings who may plausibly qualify as rightholders but who may not have the genetic basis for moral agency.
>
> (Liao 2010a, p. 168)

So, if a kitten were genetically engineered to become an agent, such a "kitten," if that is the proper term for the radically new being, would have rights. If a human being were genetically engineered not to become an agent, that human being might still have rights on other grounds.

5.1.2 Humans are Rational Animals

Many individual human beings do not function rationally, including the human embryo, the human fetus, the senile, the sleeping, the temporarily comatose, and the mentally handicapped. Such human beings cannot communicate, and they do not have conscious self-awareness. However, every single human being is nevertheless properly described as a rational being. Not a *potentially* rational being, but a currently existing *actual* rational being. This claim might be clarified by considering human anatomy. A male with testicles or a female with ovaries currently and actually (not later and potentially) possesses genital or reproductive organs. Now not every human being having reproductive organs actually reproduces. Some are too old, others too young. Some are permanently or temporarily sterile, others never have sexual intercourse. But the reproductive organs of such human beings, as well as the reproductive organs of those who do have children, are properly named and described as the reproductive or genital (ordered to generating) organs because these are the *kinds* of organs that in some circumstances perform the act which uniquely specifies them. The reproductive organs are not merely *potentially* the reproductive organs, simply because they are not functionally engaged in the act of reproducing. They *actually are* the reproductive organs. The genital organs remain genital organs even when they are not generating or are incapable of generating new life.

In the same way, every single human being *is* a rational being, even though human beings as individuals do not always function rationally. Obviously, not all human beings function rationally at any given time, but every human being is a member of a kind of being (namely human beings) who can, in certain circumstances, perform actions specifically defined as rational. In a similar way the genitals of a sterilized adult are still properly called reproductive organs (though they are no longer properly functioning reproductive organs), so too an immature human being *is* a rational being (though not yet a properly functioning rational being). The reproductive or genital organs merit a certain kind of respect (e.g., touching someone's hand is appropriate in many situations where touching the same person's genitals would not be) in virtue of the kind of organs they are even if in a given case a person's reproductive or genital organs cannot in fact (yet) generate or reproduce. Indeed, like reproductive organs, often even rational animals capable of functioning rationally are not performing their specifying activity.

To say that the human being in utero is not a rational being because he or she is not functioning rationally makes as much sense as saying that a human being is not gendered male or female unless in the act of successfully reproducing. Successful reproduction follows from the endowment (from conception) as female or male, and it is from this endowment that the sex organs emerge, secondary sex characteristics develop, and reproductive activity becomes possible. Even if a human being never performs the activity specific to being male or female (reproduction), that human being is still male or female. Even if a human being never performs the activity specific to a rational being (reasoning), that human being is still rational.

Why does *membership in a kind*—presumably a natural kind—matter so much? Why should it matter that, for instance, mentally handicapped human beings are of the same natural kind as beings such as ourselves reading this book who, by their nature, manifest the relevant property? The very genes of some human beings (such as those with grave genetic defect) guarantee a lack of capacity for rationality, so they seem by their nature non-rational. Why should species membership be morally relevant? In addition, how do we know which natural kind is the relevant one? I believe I am essentially a human animal. But I am also essentially a primate, a mammal, a vertebrate, and a living being. Which natural kind is crucial and why?

Species membership is morally relevant, argues Martha Nussbaum, because it gives us a benchmark by which to judge the flourishing of an individual member of a species (Nussbaum 2006; Anderson 2004, pp. 281–283). For example, for a human being of a certain age to be unable to read indicates a failure of that individual to flourish fully; whereas a squirrel can flourish qua squirrel without reading. Ethical decisions bear upon promoting or thwarting the flourishing of others. Since there are species-specific kinds of flourishing, the natural kind of the being in question matters ethically.

In an article devoted to exploring Martha Nussbaum's book *Hiding from Humanity*, John Haldane notices that although Nussbaum defends other vulnerable, dependent, and underdeveloped human beings, she is silent about the moral status of the unborn—though her inclusive principles and emphasis on capabilities rather than actual performative excellence would seem to suggest that the unborn should be accorded moral status and protection by law (Haldane 2008).

In addition to denying equal human moral status to the human embryo (for reasons addressed in the next chapter), Nussbaum also points out that the fetus is dependent upon one particular person, as opposed to most other vulnerable, needy, and dependent humans who can possibly be cared for by other human beings. So, the normal case of a vulnerable human being and the case of the human fetus are not alike.

Of course, we can easily imagine scenarios where only one person can care for some other human being, but in such cases we do not think that the dependent human being has thereby lost or even has been diminished in moral status. Imagine an ICU patient being cared for by hospital staff. A tyrant forces the entire staff to leave the hospital to serve injured military personnel in another location, but one doctor hides herself during the forced evacuation so as to remain behind to save the patients. In the now abandoned hospital, the patient is kept alive by the single doctor. Did the moral status of the patient change following the evacuation of the hospital staff? Would the moral status of the patient change again if several more doctors arrived at the hospital? It would seem moral status has nothing to do with whether a vulnerable human being is dependent upon many other people or only a single other person.

Strictly speaking, the unique dependency of the human fetus is only in play before viability because after viability the baby could be delivered and cared for by others. Likewise, the IVF human embryo does not depend upon any particular person but could be implanted in any one of a number of women. It is counterintuitive to hold that the IVF embryo who is not dependent on any particular woman has a greater moral status than a human fetus just prior to viability.

In any case, it is unclear why the unique dependency of the human fetus is relevant for its moral status. The human fetus is even more vulnerable, needy, and dependent than other vulnerable, needy, and dependent human beings since only one person, not a variety of persons can provide the needed care. But even confining the discussion to a pre-viable human fetus, Nussbaum has failed to address the question put to her by Haldane. If neediness, vulnerability, and dependence do not undermine moral status generally, why should the relatively greater degree of neediness, vulnerability, and dependence be relevant to the moral status of the fetus?

Others object to the view that human beings have equal basic moral status from natural capacity for rationality because some human beings have a greater capacity for rationality than others (Stretton 2008, p. 794). Human beings who are severely disabled are hardly at all ordered toward the goods of rationality. If human flourishing is important, the wrongness of taking a human life would seem to be a function of the degree to which a killing interferes with a human's flourishing. So, in cases like human mental disablement, since human flourishing is already compromised, killing such a human being would not be morally problematic.

Let me put the problem differently. On the one hand, if our moral dignity is based on the mere fact that we are all biologically human, then we can account for the moral equality of persons, but we lack an understanding of why killing is wrong. On the other hand, if what we regard as morally crucial is conceptually tied up with human flourishing or our ordering toward the goods of rationality and freedom, then we have an account that will allow us to understand why killing innocent human beings is wrong, but at the price of creating a difficulty for the equality thesis. One cannot have it both ways.

This objection rests on crucial mistakes. The first is the assumption that severely disabled human beings are not ordered toward the goods of rationality. As James Reichmann has pointed out, the human body itself differs in structure from non-human animals by being characterized by a structural openness and extreme flexibility which enables the human body, through habit and training, to properly adapt to and shape its environment far more than is possible for non-human animals (Reichmann 1985, pp. 186–189). Both instinct and physical structure limit non-human animals to a relatively smaller range of activities than human beings. The human person lives in a wild diversity of ways made possible by the mind, yes, but also by the human body's adaptability to a range of habits. The human body, even aside from the brain, is itself shaped by its intrinsic connection to reason's flexibility in the face of changing circumstances.

Furthermore, an account of human flourishing allows us to identify and bemoan human mental handicap as a painful lack of flourishing. It is in virtue of an account of species-specific flourishing that we take it as a serious loss for them and the human community that mentally handicapped human beings cannot fully flourish as the kinds of beings that they are. A mentally disabled human being and a normal hedgehog are equally incapable of exercising distinctly human reasoning and freedom, but the handicap of the human is tragic while the rational incapacity a hedgehog is inconsequential. This difference rests on the fact that the human, but not the hedgehog cannot exercise his or her species-specific form of flourishing. Since even mentally handicapped human beings share in a species-specific form of flourishing ordered to the goods of rationality and freedom, they are human persons.

By contrast, it seems wrong to say, since even mentally handicapped human beings share in a species-specific form of flourishing ordered to the goods of rationality and freedom, they have the same duties as other human persons. How can they share in the rights of human persons unless they also share in the duties of human persons?

The reason for attributing rights to these human beings but not duties is that our moral duties are always limited by what we are capable of doing. Properly understood, ought to implies can. A 1-year-old child has no duties because she is incapable of human responsibility which is generated only later through improved abilities of memory, self-control, and rationality. But a 1-year-old child—even advocates of infanticide agree—still has a right to life. In a similar way, while sleeping or temporarily unconscious we have no duties but we retain our rights. Likewise, those with debilitating conditions like strokes or brain cancer do not have moral duties permanently or temporarily if they have lost their ability to discharge their moral duties permanently or temporarily, and yet they still retain moral rights not to be killed or abused. Since we often attribute rights to human beings without also assigning them duties, we can also do so in the case of human beings in utero.

Second, the wrongness of taking a human life is not a function of *the degree* to which a killing interferes with a human's flourishing. Species-specific accounts of flourishing are relevant to determining what sorts of goods various kinds of being are ordered to and therefore to what degree they merit respect. But, for all species, it is a harm to lose the good of life, for this good is constitutive of their very selves (in addition to being a necessary condition for other aspects of flourishing). In other words, the most basic and fundamental element of the flourishing of *any* living being is *to be alive*. So, killing a being always harms that being, and the harm of killing takes away a good equally shared by all living beings—life itself. To kill a human being always harms that human being in virtue of the life he or she loses. Killing a human being undermines flourishing in the most basic and fundamental sense.

Distinction of species is also ethically relevant because we simply cannot assign moral duties based on all the unique characteristics of each animal (human or non-human) in question. As Richard Epstein put it, "Coordinating the rights and duties of countless pairs of unrelated individuals cannot rest on subtle sliding scales with uncertain substantive content. It depends on clear classifications known and observable by all" (2004, pp. 150–151). Assigning moral worth to members of species rather than to particular individuals facilitates moral judgment and provides a level standard for equal basic rights. An important objection to the view that human beings are always rational animals comes from brain transplant cases, and this objection will be examined later in this chapter.

5.1.3 The Lessons of History

That biological humanity does not depend on human choice, pluralistic consensus, or social recognition is a good thing for Jews in anti-Semitic societies, slaves dominated by slaveholders, and women not recognized by patriarchal domination. History provides strong evidence in favor of an inclusive society in which all human beings are respected as persons having dignity as opposed to an exclusive society. Indeed, when considered in light of history it seems apparent that *every single time* the performance view has been chosen over the endowment view, gross moral mistakes were made. Although the legacy of discrimination is not entirely behind us, virtually no one today (at least in the West) would publicly defend any of the applications of the performance view—slavery, misogyny, racism, sexism, anti-Catholicism, or anti-Semitism. *Every* previous division of humankind was divided into two classes by some version of performance evaluation in which one half was permitted to dispose of the other at will—men exploiting women, whites selling blacks, the young dispatching the old, the rich utilizing the poor, the healthy overpowering the sickly—and are nearly universally recognized as evil (for a contrary view, see Hoche and Binding's unfortunately influential book *Die Freigabe der Vernichtung Lebensunwertem Lebens*, 1920). Do we really have reason to believe that for the very first time in human history we are justified in treating some human beings as less than fully persons? Or will we be judged by history as just one more episode in the long line of exploitation of the powerful over the weak?

5.2 When Do Humans Begin to Exist?

Although an answer has been given to the question "is every human being a person?" it remains to be seen how this would apply to the issue of abortion. Hence, the subsidiary question: Do human beings begin to exist at conception? Again, it is helpful to clarify the nature of the question. This question is not primarily a moral question ("When does personhood begin?") but rather a scientific question ("When do human beings begin to exist?" or "Do members of the species *Homo sapiens* begin to exist at conception?"). Note too that the question is not "Do *all* human beings begin to exist at conception?" Certainly it is *logically* possible for a human being to come into existence without fertilization of an egg by a sperm. Greek mythology portrays Athena (admittedly more goddess than woman) as springing fully grown from the head of Zeus. Aristophanes in Plato's *Symposium* imagines the original human beings as circular people who roll around like tires and were fashioned from the sun, moon, and earth. These beings become human as we are currently through an act of punishment from Zeus splitting them in two and then arranging sexual intercourse as an imperfect attempt to recreate a lost unity. Contemporary science also holds out the possibility of human life beginning without union of sperm and egg by means of cloning. Indeed, the birth of a human being brought into existence without fertilization of egg and sperm was announced on December 26, 2002. On this day, a statement was issued to major news networks that a woman, sponsored by the Raelian cult (who believe that human life arose from cloned aliens), had given birth to the first cloned human being, a baby girl named "Eve." At the time of my writing, this claim has yet to be independently confirmed, it may be that someone, somewhere in the future will give birth to a cloned child. Even before this took place, the phenomenon of the natural cloning known as monozygotic twinning (one human embryo splitting and giving rise to identical twins) shows that at least some human beings do not begin to exist at conception. So the question at hand here is not whether *all* human beings begin to exist at conception (they clearly don't) but rather whether *some* human beings, in fact the vast majority of human beings, begin to exist at conception.

This is a biological question, and we could quote here, page after page, numerous biologists, scientists, and physicians who have provided clear answers to this question. In the interest of space, let's consider only three texts (noted earlier by Lee 1996):

> The formation, maturation, and meeting of a male and female sex cell are all preliminary to their actual union into a combined cell, or zygote, which definitely marks the beginning of a new individual. This penetration of the ovum by spermatozoon, and the coming together and pooling of their respective nuclei, constitutes the process of fertilization.
>
> (Arey 1974, p. 55)

> Zygote. This cell is the beginning of a human being. It results from the fertilization of an ovum by a sperm. The expression "fertilized ovum" refers to the zygote.
>
> (Moore 1987, p. 9)

> Embryonic life commences with fertilization, and hence the beginning of that process may be taken as the point of departure of stage I.
>
> (Larsen 1993, p. 19)

Indeed, summarizing hours of testimony, the official U.S. Senate report on Senate Bill 158, the "Human Life Bill," stated:

> Physicians, biologists, and other scientists agree that conception marks the beginning of the life of a human being—a being that is alive and is a member of the human species. There is overwhelming agreement on this point in countless medical, biological, and scientific writings.
>
> (cited by Alcorn 2000, p. 55)

Patrick Lee quotes a number of scientists, some of whose words appear above, and then goes on to suggest reasons why it makes sense to hold that fertilization marks the start of a new human life (1996, p. 71). First, to claim that the zygote is not the same organism as the fetus, newborn, or child requires positing significant additional changes without need or cause. No outside agency is present changing the newly conceived organism into something else, but rather the human embryo is self-developing towards functional rationality. Speaking analogously, the human embryo is therefore not merely a detailed blueprint of the house that will be built but a tiny house that constructs itself larger and more complex through its active self-development towards maturity.

Second, Lee notes a radical discontinuity between sperm and egg, on the one hand, and the human zygote on the other:

> The actual coming to be of an organism cannot be a gradual process. As Aristotle noted long ago, there are no degrees of being a substance or a concrete thing: one either is or is not a horse, one either is or is not an amoeba. Even if the changes which lead to the coming to be of a new organism may be gradual, the transition to actually being one must be instantaneous, and therefore involve a discontinuity. . . . Fertilization is a radical discontinuity in a series of events in which it does not seem possible to place necessary discontinuity anywhere else.
>
> (1996, p. 71)

The radical discontinuity occurs at the completion of fertilization because it is then that a being with 46 chromosomes, a being which previously did not exist, first comes into existence and the individual gametes, the sperm having 23 and the ovum having 23, cease to exist.

A human embryo is properly classified as an individual human being rather than a collection of human cells, a member of the kind *Homo sapiens* rather than simply a "heap" of cells of human origin (Condic 2003, p. 52). A shaving of your skin may contain living human cells, but the skin shavings as a group are just an uncoordinated heap, whereas you are a self-developing and self-integrated whole whose various parts (skin, eyes, arms, blood) serve the whole. Such skin cells are merely parts of a human being without a dynamic, intrinsic orientation to develop towards maturity in the human species. By contrast, the human embryo is a whole, complete organism, a living individual human being whose cells work together in a coordinated effort of self-development towards maturity. If all human beings are persons, then the human embryo is a person.

5.3 The Constitutive Property Argument

To summarize the chapter thus far, if all human beings are persons and if human beings begin to exist at conception, then persons begin to exist at conception. But let us consider another approach to the question at hand which arrives at the same conclusion. Slightly altering the formulation of Boonin (2003, p. 52), one could also make a "constitutive property" argument for personhood in the following way:

P1: If an individual being has a constitutive property at one point in time, then it has that property at every point in its existence.
P2: You are the same individual living being or organism as the fetus from which you developed.
P3: You are a human person constitutively.
C: The zygote from which you developed was a human person.

Of course, there is nothing particular about this argument that makes it apply only to you and not every other human being, so if this argument is sound, it would show that every human fetus is also a human person. Since a human being in later stages of life are less contentiously held to be persons than the human fetus, *a fortiori*, if even a human fetus is a person, then every other human being is also a person.

Let's start with what is most easily shown. P1 (if an individual being has a constitutive or essential property at one point in time, then it has that property at every point in its existence) is true by definition, since what X has constitutively must always be a characteristic of X, otherwise it is not a *constitutive* characteristic, but an accidental characteristic. Triangles constitutively have three sides, and if a figure does not have three sides, then this figure is not (or is no longer) a triangle. So if a figure is a triangle, then it must have three sides from the very beginning of its being a triangle until the end of its being a triangle, since having three sides is a *constitutive characteristic* of any triangle. That the triangle's sides are of equal measure is not a constitutive characteristic of a triangle, but an accidental characteristic of a triangle. Some triangles have sides of equal measure; others do not.

So P1 is true, but what about P2, are you the same individual living being as the fetus from which you developed? Before arguing for this premise I should also make clear that accepting this premise does not of itself entail the impermissibility of feticide. Recognizing continuity before and after birth does not in itself lead to a pro-life conclusion. As Boonin notes in his book *A Defense of Abortion*:

> In the top drawer of my desk I keep another picture of [my son] Eli. This picture was taken September 7, 1993, 24 weeks before he was born. The sonogram image is murky, but it reveals clearly enough a small head tilted back slightly, and an arm raised up and bent, with the hand pointing back towards the face and the thumb extended out toward the mouth. There is no doubt in my mind that this picture, too, shows the same little boy at a very early stage in his physical development. And there is no question that the position I defend in this book entails that [it] would have been morally permissible to end his life at this point.
>
> (2003, p. xiv)

The truth of the premise that you are the same individual living being as the fetus from which you developed is a matter of observation and scientific data. You now, you at ten years old, you at ten days following birth, you ten days after conception and you at all stages of your life in between stand in bodily continuity. We also can have the experience of watching the development of a single human being through various stages after birth and through maturity. If wombs had windows, we would be able to watch this one human being grow throughout various stages of development before birth as well. Pregnant women and their physicians can have this experience at least partially in charting the course of a pregnancy. The being whose existence became known through a pregnancy test is the same being whose ultrasound picture was on the refrigerator, who stirred in womb, and who was finally born. If a stranger attacks the mother and permanently damages the human fetus within her, then throughout all future phases of life from cradle through kindergarten and from adulthood to grave, this human being will suffer on account of the damage suffered while in utero.

McMahan argues against P2 by claiming that you and I are "embodied minds" that began to exist when our brains gained the capacity for consciousness and cease to exist when our brain loses this capacity

(McMahan 2002, p. 69; Savulescu 2002). With our neural capacity, we come into existence and cease to exist—we are embodied minds. So abortions prior to the emergence of the capacity for consciousness, the vast majority of abortions, do not kill a being like you or me, for we are essentially embodied minds.

There are really two different, opposing standards at work here, each with its own difficulty. McMahan summarizes the two different theses in the following sentences: "We continue to exist as long as those areas of the brain in which consciousness is realized retain the capacity for consciousness. When the capacity is irreversibly lost, we cease to exist" (2005, pp. 1–2).

The first sentence claims that actual capacity for consciousness is needed for our identity. A difficulty with this view is the possibility of our brains losing neural capacity and gaining it back. For centuries, serious damage to the hip meant an end to a person's capacity to walk. Now, we have full or partial hip replacement re-enabling those who had lost the capacity to walk. We cannot currently perform surgery to repair injured parts of the brain, but it is in principle possible that lack of neural capacity could be restored for the victim of accident or disease. If this takes place, and if actual capacity for consciousness is necessary for our identity, then we could come into existence and leave existence many times over, as often as we were injured and had brain surgery to restore neural capacity. We have the episodic problem in spades.

But perhaps actual neural capacity is not needed. According to the second standard, we die when neural capacity is *irreversibly* lost. Actual neural capacity need not be present (the person's brain may be so damaged as to destroy this capacity) so long as neural capacity could be actualized in the future. This view preserves the identity of the person in the temporary coma whose brain can be restored to neural capacity. However, on this second view, the human being in a temporary coma and the human embryo alike are beings that have not permanently lost the capacity for consciousness. Indeed, in some cases, this capacity may be actualized more quickly and easily in the human embryo than in the coma victim. McMahan's account of human identity as constituted by the capacity to support consciousness mirrors the weaknesses of the account of personhood as the capacity for self-awareness discussed earlier in section 2.4.

Peter Singer also disputes P2 by suggesting that you and I are not the same beings that we were earlier in our existence, at the embryonic, fetal, and newborn stages of human life. If Singer is correct, then who I am, as a person, is constituted by overlapping mental links of memory (Singer 2000, p. 136). In other words, my continuity as a person is not a matter of biological continuity but of mental continuity—a continuity of memory. Since this obviously does not stretch back to conception, I am not the same being who was conceived by my mother and father.

Singer's conception of personal identity presupposes that "I" am only my conceptions, memories, or thoughts, not my bodily existence. As expressed by Ronald Dworkin, my "personal life" as a being due respect differs from my "biological life" as a corporeal organism (1994). Indeed, we know we are the same person each day not because we wake up, look in the mirror, and see the same body, but because our desires, memories, expectations, and mental life are continuous from one day to the next. It is possible to imagine scenarios of waking up in another person's body or with another person's memories. In these science fiction worlds, you might wake up tomorrow, look in the mirror, and see the face and body of Arnold Schwarzenegger staring back. He might wake up and find himself looking in the mirror at what you now take to be your body. On this view of personal identity, my body, which predates my conceptions, memories, or thoughts, is something else that does not count as "me."

There are many reasons to reject such views of personal identity, in part because the evidence to which they appeal seems to point in the opposite direction. If you were to wake up tomorrow with a different personality and memories, others would not in fact conclude that you were a different person but rather that you are the same person as before, but a person suffering from mental illness of some kind. In actual practice, we do identify various persons by their bodily identities and not by their mental contents.

If the account of identity offered by Singer, Dworkin, and McMahan were true, in assaulting a person's body through rape, torture, or mutilation, the attacker does not really directly harm a *person* (which is merely the ghost in the machine so to speak), but directly harms what might be considered the person's property or the human organism he or she occupies. Rape, torture, and mutilation only indirectly harm persons by interfering with the plans and goals of the conscious mind. However, if you chop off my arm, isn't it accurate to say you have harmed *me*, not simply something I own and make use of? Slashing the tire of my car is one thing; slashing my Achilles tendon is quite another. Rape, torture, and mutilation directly harm persons in addition to interfering with the plans and desires of a conscious mind. A rapist violates an unconscious woman even if she does not remember it afterwards, even if the rape never impinges on her conscious mind. Intuitions such as these point to the conclusion that we are—rather than simply make use of—our bodies.

This conception of personal identity is also supported by consideration of our sensate life (Lee 1998). Sensing is a bodily act. We hear, see, touch, taste, and smell only in so far as we are bodily beings, making use of bodily organs. Without eyes, without the body, there is no sight and the same is true of other senses. Now, we regularly think and communicate such as follows: "I see the tree and feel the sun's rays." In doing so, *we* are making a judgment about the world. Now it is the same *we* that senses and that makes the intellectual judgment, so *we* are both bodily and intellectual beings, indeed intellectual by means of our bodily senses. We are not purely "spiritual beings" making use of physical bodies, but bodily beings who are intellectual.

Singer's conception of personal identity leads to other difficulties as well. For instance, no man could say, "I was circumcized," unless his circumcision took place after he began to remember. "When were you born?" asks the shopkeeper checking the age of someone wanting to buy alcohol. "Well, actually, *I* wasn't born. In fact, *you* were not born either. Indeed, I don't know a single person who was born." The shopkeeper would have reason for thinking someone giving such an answer had already had quite enough to drink.

Others have objected that the mental continuity theory of identity is circular for it presupposes what needs to be explained. Is Katie the same person as Gracie? Well, if Katie and Gracie have the same memories, according to the psychological theory of identity the answer will be "yes." But of course some people have false memories, so Katie might *believe* she remembers doing what Gracie did but she might be mistaken (because of hypnosis, drug use, mental error, or some other cause). How then do we distinguish false memories from true memories? Well, true memories are ones that really happened to the person in question, and false memories are ones that did not really happen to the person in question. If Gracie remembers going to the Grand Canyon, and in fact Gracie has never been to the Grand Canyon, her memories are false. So, we need to know the *identity of the person in question* to find out if the memories are true or false. But the very purpose of the mental continuity theory of identity is to figure out "who is who," but the theory cannot do this without already knowing who is who.

Even if the circularity problem could be resolved, another *prima facie* difficulty with mental continuity theory of identity remains, namely, the copy objection. Imagine you could copy the memories of Kelly in Kansas City, a process that destroys the human being with which Kelly was associated. You then put these memories and mental contents into two different human beings (who have had their memories erased), one in Los Angeles and the other in New York City. If the mental continuity theory were true, then *both* of these human beings would be the same person, Kelly. One person, the same person, would simultaneously be in Los Angeles and not be in Los Angeles: a contradiction. (Whether the circularity and copy objections are also *ultima facie* successful remains a matter of debate. For more objections and responses to the mental continuity theory of personal identity, as well as alternative accounts, see Feser 2005 and Olson 1997a.)

Michael Tooley imagines a variety of examples which lead to a rejection of P2 and are meant to point to the conclusion that we are not rational animals, the same living organism as the human fetus from which we developed (Tooley, Wolf-Devine, Devine, & Jaggar 2009, pp. 53–58). Let's say you had to choose between the following two scenarios. In scenario one, your body is completely destroyed except for your upper brain, which is transplanted into another body allowing a psychological continuity of your consciousness, thoughts, beliefs, desires and plans. In scenario two, your upper brain is completely destroyed but the rest of your body remains. Which scenario would you choose? Most people would preserve their upper brain. Tooley's conclusion is that this intuition is explained by the fact that we are not essentially rational animals or human organisms, since we would prefer to have the organism with which we are associated destroyed rather than have our upper brain destroyed.

Tooley also imagines cases of transplantation of upper brains among various bodies. Let's say the upper brain of Mary is switched with the upper brain of John, so that all Mary's beliefs, memories, personality traits, and psychological capacities are now associated with John's body, and all John's beliefs, memories, personality traits, and psychological capacities are now associated with Mary's body. If the organism view were correct, reasons Tooley, we would have to say that after the transplant, the body originally belonging to Mary is still really Mary, even though this body is now associated with the beliefs, memories, and personality traits of John. The truth, in Tooley's view, is that Mary now has a different animal body, the body formerly used by John. So, what makes Mary remain Mary is the continuity of her psychological characteristics over time in whatever body she may find herself. Thus, it is incorrect to say that we are essentially rational animals or human organisms. Do these examples show that human beings are not rational animals?

Tooley's first example confuses the question of identity with the question of what we have a greater interest in preserving. If you had to choose between having your entire arm cut off, leaving just a thumb reattached where your arm formerly was, or having a thumb cut off, leaving the rest of your arm intact, which would you choose? Well, obviously you'd choose to have just a finger cut off, but it hardly follows from that preference that your thumb isn't really a part of your body or that your body does not (now) include your finger. In other words, your thumb is no less a part of you than your arm, but it is a less important part of you in terms of your overall well-being. Similarly, most people would prefer both legs destroyed rather than both lungs, even though the legs are a greater part of us in terms of mass. In like manner, if faced with a choice between having the rest of your body destroyed while preserving your brain or having your brain destroyed while preserving the rest of your body, we would choose the brain over the rest of the body, but it does not necessarily follow that "I" am simply my brain. The intuition that we would choose our brains might reflect a judgment about the relative value of various parts of our bodies, rather than a judgment about what essentially constitutes us. The rest of your body is no less a part of you (indeed it is the greater part of you in terms of mass) than your brain, even though your brain (in virtue of its role in your thinking) is the more important part of you. Tooley's objection trades on a confusion between what is more *valuable* to you and what *is* you, a confusion identified several years ago by Derek Parfit (1987). As David Hershenov describes (but not endorses) this response, "we are misled into thinking that we would be transplanted because of mistaken belief that identity is what matters to us in survival" (2008, p. 483). We can account for the choice of brain over the rest of the body without assuming a psychological view of personal identity or that we are really just our brains.

Further, the transplant objection may not undermine the view that we are rational animals, for perhaps we can construe the brain, or even the upper brain, as the smallest possible reduction of a human organism. Eric Olson suggests this interpretation of the transplant case,

> The surgeons do not move your cerebrum from one animal to another in the transplant story. Rather, one animal has its parts cut away until it is the size of a cerebrum. It is then moved across the room and given a new complement of parts. The animal into which your cerebrum is implanted then presumably ceases to exist.
>
> (Olson 2008)

In this interpretation of the transplant objection, we can grant the intuition that "we" go with our brains so to speak, but still maintain that we are rational animals, albeit in the transplant case radically mutilated animals missing most of our bodies. In other words, if we were to assume that the smallest possible reduction of a human being would be to the size of the upper brain, then if we moved the upper brain, it would still be a human organism that we move, albeit a radically impaired organism until implanted in another body whose organs would then take over the functions formerly exercised by the previous body.

David Hershenov points out another difficulty for Tooley's view that we are our brains.

> So if we are to understand the person as the subject minimally sufficient for thought, perhaps then by analogy, we should understand the organism as the subject minimally sufficient for life. But does this mean then that the organism only derivatively possesses feet and kidneys? That's preposterous. The organism is much larger than the brain, it is just that it can be reduced in size to the bare minimum essential for life. Thus it would be a mistake to confuse the organism with the smallest possible form that it can take. Have McMahan and Persson made a similar mistake in regards to the person? If so, a person could then be six feet and two hundred pounds, though

that same person could be reduced in size to just essential cerebral parts.

(2005, p. 32)

Even if an organism could be radically reduced in size, it does not follow that prior to its reduction it is "really" or in essence only the smallest size it could possibly be reduced to and survive.

However, the view that you really are just your cerebrum also leads to bizarre and counter-intuitive conclusions. If this were true, as Hershenov points out,

> The average adult person is not really somewhere between 5 and 6 feet tall, 100 and 200 pounds. Instead, most people consist of just a few inches and pounds of grey matter. Taking this claim literally means that a person couldn't have pains in his feet.
>
> (2005, p. 31)

If we are nothing but our brains, then we never see persons (unless we're present for brain surgery), we could not normally distinguish one person from another by appearance even if we did see persons, and we never kiss or have been kissed by a person.

Tooley makes use of far-fetched cases, cases which are not only impossible to accomplish now but may never be physically possible. But such fantasy examples also cause trouble for the other main accounts of personal identity. Imagine cases in which there is fission of the brain itself, so that one hemisphere of your cerebrum goes to one body and the other hemisphere goes to another body. Eric Olson points out the troubles that arise from such examples.

> The two recipients—call them Lefty and Righty—will each be psychologically continuous with you. The Psychological Approach as I have stated it implies that any future being who is psychologically continuous with you must be you. It follows that you are Lefty and also that you are Righty. But that cannot be: Lefty and Righty are two, and one thing cannot be numerically identical with two things. Suppose Lefty is hungry at a time when Righty isn't. If you are Lefty, you are hungry at that time. If you are Righty, you aren't. If you are Lefty *and* Righty, you are both hungry and not hungry at once: a contradiction.
>
> (2008)

The same problem arises for the embodied mind account, since the embodied mind is found in two hemispheres which, if we admit bizarre examples, could be transplanted into different bodies giving rise to Lefty and Righty.

The defender of the psychological approach could say at this point that a person X is identical to a later person Y just in case Y is *fully* psychologically continuous with X. This doesn't seem *ad hoc*; and it would allow the defender of the psychological approach to deny that you are both Lefty and Righty (you wouldn't be identical to either one, since neither is fully psychologically continuous with you). However, in the brain fission cases as imagined in copying cases, both Lefty and Righty are *both* fully psychologically continuous with you, so this response does not alleviate the problem.

Advocates of the psychological continuity view or the embodied mind view will characteristically respond to cases of fission by adding a "non-branching" clause to their account, such that their view is true so long as there is no branching of the psychological continuity between two (or more) different recipients. But, if adding a non-branching clause is not excluded as *ad hoc*, then there is no reason that advocates of the rational animal view cannot also add a non-branching clause with respect to the branching of the brain from the rest of the body of the human animal. So, the move that shores up the psychological continuity view ends up also shoring up the rational animal view against brain transplant examples.

The non-branching view has additional troubles, as Olson notes:

> This proposal, the "non-branching view," has the surprising consequence that if your brain is divided, you will survive if only one half is preserved, but you will die if both halves are. That is just the opposite of what most of us expect: if your survival depends on the functioning of your brain (because that is what underlies psychological continuity), then the more of that organ we preserve, the greater ought to be your chance of surviving. In fact, the non-branching view implies you would perish if one of your hemispheres were transplanted and the other left in place: you can survive hemispherectomy only if the excised hemisphere is immediately destroyed.
>
> (2008)

This means that if one of your hemispheres were successfully implanted, and you did not know what happened to the other hemisphere, then you would not know whether or not you survived, even though you (in some sense) would be the one thinking about the question of whether you survived:

> Faced with the prospect of having one of your hemispheres transplanted, there would seem to be no reason to prefer that the other be destroyed. Most of us would rather have both preserved, even if they go into different heads. Yet on the non-branching view that is to prefer death over continued existence.
>
> (Olson 2008)

Adding a clause about branching, in other words, does not solve the problems raised by fission.

Of course, one could say that severing the distinct hemispheres of the brain and placing each half in another organism is physically impossible and so irrelevant. One could also say that our intuitions about severing the distinct hemispheres of the brain and placing each half in another organism are irrelevant. Since we have never actually encountered such bizarre transformations, we might claim that "our ignorance about what actually happens in these cases jeopardizes the theoretical relevance of fission scenarios" (Korfmacher 2006). But if we are going to rule out far-fetched counter examples to the psychological continuity account on the basis of physical impossibility or on the basis of the unreliability of our intuitions about bizarre cases, then we equally have to rule out such examples, such as cerebrum switches between human organisms, as possible objections to the view that we are rational animals.

Jeff McMahan raises an objection to the view that we are rational animals that does not rely on science fiction (McMahan 2002, p. 35). In cases of Dicephalus conjoined twins, there is one body shared by two heads. For example, the Hensel twins, Abigail and Brittany, were two persons, but only one shared organism. It is possible for one person to die, but the other survive. Let's say Brittany gets struck in the head with a baseball flying at high velocity, but Abigail does not. Brittany dies from the injury but the animal organism—now connected only to Abigail—continues to live. This case shows that Brittany was not a rational animal because the rational animal survived her death. Since we are the same kind of being as Brittany, we are also not rational animals.

Matthew Liao notes a problem with this argument.

> In response to the Dicephalus Case, it may be said that there are in fact two organisms, although they may not be completely independent organisms. In most cases of dicephalus, it is possible to identify functioning organs for two organisms. For example, in McMahan's example of Abigail and Brittany Hensel, each twin has her own stomach and heart; they have distinct brainstems and distinct spines that are only joined at the hips; and they have partially distinct organs that are united. This suggests that in fact, there are two organisms here although they are not fully independent organisms.
>
> (2006b, p. 340)

Imagination can suggest cases where conjoined twins are even more closely intertwined than were Abigail and Brittany, but even these cases suggest that "there are two capacities for coordinating various life processes, and that therefore, there are two organisms" (Liao 2006b, p. 341).

Liao also lodges a powerful objection to the psychological account of personal identity, probably the chief rival of the view that human beings are rational animals. Liao notes that Dissociative Identity Disorder (DID) or Multiple Personality Disorder, with up to 16 different sets of memories and experiences would constitute 16 different persons making use or associated with one human organism. But then to cure such a disorder—by destroying the various extra personalities—would be the same morally as killing 15 human persons (Liao 2006b, p. 342). However, in alleviating multiple personality disorder, a doctor cures, not kills. So, our personal identity is not merely a matter of memories, beliefs, and desires. The upshot of these discussions is that Tooley's fantasy transplant examples need not undermine the view that we are rational animals, but real life examples do undermine the psychological continuity view of personal identity.

So if P1 and P2 are true, all that remains to be shown is P3, you are a person constitutively or essentially. If one defines a person as an individual substance of rational nature (Boethius) or as a being endowed with freedom even if not exercising it (Kant), then P3 would be true by definition since what is by nature or endowment is constitutively an aspect of the being in question. If one defines a person as a member of a kind of being that is rational, then it is also the case that you are a personal constitutively. A constitutive characteristic is the contrary of all that is conventional, superficial, or learned. But being a member of the species *Homo sapiens* is just such a characteristic for it is not a matter of convention (like which side of the road to drive on), nor is it a superficial characteristic (like length of hair), nor does it arise from training (we don't learn how to be a member of the species *Homo sapiens*). Being a member of a kind of being (human) is a characteristic such that to cease being a member of this kind is for *you* to cease to exist. You can change in countless ways, but if you ceased being a human being and became, say, 10,000 bits of plant fertilizer, then *you* would be no longer living but dead. Indeed, if anything is a constitutive characteristic of you, being a human being is. I can get a sex change operation and live to tell; I cannot get a species change operation and remain alive. So, if a person is a member of a kind of being that is rational, and if being a kind of being is a constitutive property, then every person is constitutively a person.

We have reason to endorse the idea that we are persons constitutively as a means of avoiding the episodic problem mentioned earlier. If we are persons constitutively, then we do not have to worry about losing our rights, gaining them back, and losing them again. We have rights so long as we are alive.

A metaphysical problem may seem to arise here. Are "person" and "human being" the same sort of properties? "Human being" is the substance sortal to which I belong, and to which I must always belong as long as I exist. So, "person" cannot also be a substance sortal of that sort since one and the same being cannot belong to two different substance sortals. So the kind of property that "person" is must not be a substance sortal but rather a phase sortal, a category like adolescent that one enters into and then can also leave while remaining substantially the same being. To be human and to be a person cannot therefore both be constitutive properties but rather are two different sorts of concepts.

To answer such an objection, it is important to remember that although one cannot belong to two different substance sortals, it does not follow that being a person must be a phase sortal rather than a constitutive property. Similarly, all human beings are animals as a constitutive aspect of being human, and this constitutive property is shared by other beings as well. In other terminology, one could say that "animal" is the larger genus to which "human" belongs. In like manner, to be human is to have a nature ordered to rationality. To flourish as a human being, and this is true for all human beings, involves making use of practical and theoretical reasoning. There may very well be other beings who enjoy a rational nature, so simply having a rational nature and this alone does not define humans as humans. Thus, this account of personhood is not "speciesism," for in principle any number of species other than humans could be persons. Yet each and every human has rational nature just as each and every human has an animal body as a constitutive property, an aspect of what they are essentially but not the fullness of what they are essentially, nor something that is necessarily possessed only by members of that kind. If one wanted to speak precisely, one might even contrast a constitutive property, an aspect of what one is essentially, with an essential property, which might be said to be had by all those who share the same essence and possessed only those who share the same essence, such as human nature for human beings.

In any case, Boonin provides two arguments against the proposition that you are constitutively a person, by arguing that accepting P3 has implications that many people, regardless of their views on abortion, would find unacceptable, namely that human beings in irreversible comas have the same right to life as you or me and that capital punishment is always wrong (Boonin 2003, p. 55; Marquis 2007, p. 396). Accepting P3 commits one to certain views about euthanasia, physician assisted suicide, or treating human beings in permanent comas that would be either questionable, unacceptable, or at the very least inconsistent with the views of many who oppose feticide. We could call this the "over commitment" objection to P3.

The over-commitment objection to P3 would not trouble all critics of abortion, since many opponents of abortion are also opposed to euthanasia. Where he sees a difficulty, they would see consistency. Indeed, many who would describe themselves as pro-choice about abortion as well as the law in most countries do not endorse direct euthanasia. If we take the law to be revelatory of common intuitions, then since most countries and states forbid intentionally killing PVS patients or anencephalic infants, common intuition must also hold that these acts are morally wrong.

Is it true that human beings in a PVS state have no rights? Imagine Jennifer Aniston falls, hits the back of her head, and slips into PVS state. That night in the hospital, a janitor comes into her room, locks the door, and has sexual intercourse with her. If human beings in a PVS state do not have basic rights, then they cannot have their rights to bodily integrity violated by rape. But everyone agrees that an unconscious human being can be raped; the length of time the victim is unconscious is irrelevant to whether it is rape. So, unconscious human beings, even human beings who will remain unconscious until death, do have rights—including the right not to be raped and *a fortiori* the right to life.

In any event, how to handle cases of irreparably brain-damaged adult human beings in complete and irreversible comas is hardly an intuitively clear matter to begin with, so to appeal to such cases in building an argument for abortion is to defend the controversial with the equally or more controversial (*obscurum per obscurius*).

Even so, the constitutive property argument does not *necessarily* and without further considerations lead to the conclusion that a being in a permanent coma or a brain-dead human being has the same right to life as you or me. If one accepts brain death or upper brain death as the criterion for the death of a human being, then what was a human being would, in such a state, be considered dead even if the corpse were in some respects functioning as it formerly did. Incontrovertibly dead bodies may on occasion twitch with death tremors. So the fact that some or even many bodily systems of a corpse still operate does not necessarily mean that a human being is alive. If a being in a permanent coma is considered brain dead or upper brain dead, and *if* the death of the whole brain or upper brain is considered legally and morally the death of a human being, then such dead human beings do not have a right to life even if various bodily activities continue. So, one could hold both that persons are persons constitutively and that, following brain death or upper brain death, the physical remains of what was once a human person does not have a right to life.

A critic might argue that if brain death really counts as death, then why should the human fetus prior to the development of the brain also not be considered dead? As indicated earlier (section 4.1.6), even if one accepts neurological criteria as the basis for determining death, an important difference between the human fetus and the case of brain death would be that of irreversibility. In brain death, brain function is not irreversibly lost, a temporary loss is not considered brain death. A brain dead patient has irreversibly lost neurological function; a human fetus has not irreversibly lost neurological function but will, if all goes well, function like the rest of us.

Even if comatose patients are considered living human beings, it would not necessarily follow, in one sense, that this human being has the same right to life as you or I. Such a human being has a right to life equal to you or me in the sense that he or she has a right not to be intentionally killed. But it does not follow from an equal right not to be intentionally killed that each person has an equal right to receive the same medical treatments. In other words, some treatments that would be appropriate to give to someone in a temporary coma may not be appropriate to give to the person in a permanent coma, because though such treatments would be of tremendous benefit to the person in the temporary coma, they may be of relatively little benefit to the person in a permanent coma. What treatments should be given is a matter of prudential judgment and should take into accounts both the burdens and the benefits of treatment. Assessing the burdens and benefits of treatment may be importantly different in cases of temporary versus permanent comas. In this imprecise sense of a right to life, the right to life of those in a permanent coma differs significantly from the right to life of those who will recover from comas. In Kantian terms, our imperfect duties to benefit others are not exactly alike but must take into account various circumstances even though our perfect duties not to intentionally harm others is alike for all human beings.

Let's suppose that these two responses are mistaken. It would still not *necessarily* follow from holding that persons are persons constitutively that a person in a permanent coma has the same right to life as you and me if one understood the right to life as an alienable right. I have an alienable right to property I own, which means that I can give up my right to this property if I choose, for example, by giving it away as a gift. Inalienable rights, on the other hand, cannot be "waived" in the same way. If liberty is an inalienable right, then any contract I enter into to make myself (or another) a slave is invalid even if I (or the other) want to become a slave. If the right to life is understood as an alienable right, say a right that one can waive at least in extreme circumstances, then persons could waive their right not to be killed and still remain constitutively persons. (I add "extreme circumstances" to exclude those who would commit suicide for frivolous reasons, such as a teenage brokenheartedness.) If you or I are not in extreme circumstances, then perhaps we cannot waive our right to life. However, unlike a depressed lovesick teenager, a person in a permanent coma is in an extreme circumstance. A human being in a permanent coma obviously cannot give consent while in the coma to be killed, but consent may be given through a living will, the decision of one previously granted power of attorney, or through proxy consent. If consent is given on behalf of the one in a permanent coma, and if the right to life is an alienable right not an inalienable right, then the right to life of a person would not be violated if the person in a coma were intentionally killed. Of course, the right to life may very well be an inalienable right, and there are many other moral considerations that must be taken into account in treating the case of euthanasia or physician-assisted suicide (for more on the topic, see Hendin 1998).

My point is not to defend the idea that the right to life is an alienable right, or that neocortical death should be defined as death or that human beings in permanent comas have a different right to life than human beings in temporary comas. Rather, these remarks are simply meant to indicate that accepting that every person is a person constitutively does not *necessarily* commit one to any given position on euthanasia or physician-assisted suicide or the treatment of those in permanent comas.

What of the other difficulty raised? Must those who accept that persons are persons constitutively also believe that capital punishment is always wrong? Indeed, since persons also enjoy the right to liberty and property, the constitutive personhood argument would also be the abolition of all fines and imprisonment as well. Constitutive personhood and criminal punishment are irreconcilably opposed according to the objection.

In fact, punishment in itself is not necessarily a denial of personhood. Application of retributive justice, giving to each what is due, actually recognizes and reaffirms the personhood of the one being punished. Although the ancients put inanimate objects on trial and punished them, we do not. We only put on trial and punish persons because only persons enjoy freedom in such a way that they may be held responsible for their actions. The ontology of a person gives rise to freedom, and freedom gives rise to responsibility. Recognition of this responsibility, by reward or by punishment, is therefore *an affirmation of personhood*. If we were to let criminals like elderly mafia dons or Nazi concentration camp officers "off the hook" with no punishment whatsoever since they no longer posed a threat to society, we would be acting on the same principle that they did: some human beings should be treated as less than persons. We would be failing to take their human responsibility seriously, and we in fact would be responding to them as we might respond to a tree or a fire that had caused human misery. Punishments of various kinds, including imprisonment, fines, and the death penalty, need not therefore be a rejection of the personhood of the one punished, indeed *just penalties* of all kinds affirm the personhood of the one punished.

Although retributive punishment and constitutive personhood are compatible, there is a debate about how to conceptualize the relationship between the two. According to one account of the relationship of personhood and punishment, a criminal deserving of punishment has waived the right to life, liberty, or property as the case may be. According to another account, a person retains their rights, but these rights have built-in exceptions for just punishment. The right to life is the right not to be intentionally killed unless duly convicted of a serious crime. Finally, even if one understood the right to life to be the right not to be intentionally killed as a means or as an end, according to some theorists, capital punishment would not violate this norm if the act chosen of itself instantiates the good of retributive justice, using the death of the other neither as a means or an end (Finnis 1991, p. 80).

In all these accounts, the constitutive personhood argument does not entail that no punishment, capital or otherwise, may ever be given to a person, indeed it suggests the opposite. The ideal of justice, giving to each person what is due, suggests that the innocent and guilty merit different treatment precisely as a response to their personhood. Of course, capital punishment might be wrong for other reasons, but it does not follow necessarily from the constitutive personhood of all human beings that capital punishment is always wrong.

Even if it were true that one would have to oppose euthanasia and capital punishment in order for the constitutive property argument to work, this might not necessarily be a problem. Advocates of what is sometimes called the "consistent life ethic" or "seamless garment" would see opposition to all three kinds of killing not as a problem but rather as consistency. They oppose all abortion, all capital punishment, and all euthanasia because they oppose all intentional killing of human beings (see, for example, Grisez 1970). But even if the consistent life ethic is correct, much work must be done to move from P3, you are a person constitutively, to any particular view about these other "life" issues, including euthanasia, physician assisted suicide, treating human beings in permanent comas, and capital punishment. Therefore, the over commitment objection to P3 fails.

In sum, the constitutive property argument shows that every human fetus is a person. If an individual being has a constitutive property at one point in time, then it has that property at every point in its existence. You are a person constitutively, ontologically. Furthermore, you are the same individual living human being as the fetus from which you developed. Thus, it follows that the fetus from which you developed was a person, and, since nothing in the argument depends on any of your unique individual characteristics, this holds also for every other human fetus. All human beings, from the zygotic to the geriatric, enjoy the same fundamental rights, including, most fundamentally, the right to life. However, it is important to consider serious objections raised to this position, especially in terms of the personhood of the human embryo, so it is these arguments that are the focus in the next chapter.

6 Does the Human Embryo Have Rights?

Although the idea that all human beings are fundamentally equal has certainly been criticized, since we have already examined many such critiques (e.g., Tooley, Singer, Warren, Engelhardt, Boonin), here the focus will be on several major objections to the view that the human embryo is a person, a being due fundamental respect. Although most abortions take place eight weeks or more after conception, after the human fetus has a beating heart, an individual blood type, and the ability to suck his or her thumb, the issue of the personhood of the early embryo has particular relevance for certain forms of chemical abortion, the most famous of which is RU-486, a method now used for approximately 6% of all abortions. Even aside from debates about abortion, the human embryo's moral status has tremendous import for discussions about embryonic stem cell research.

The most important arguments against the embryo being a human person include the following.

First, although there is no momentous change at each tiny development of an acorn into an oak tree, still it would be erroneous to claim that an acorn *is* an oak tree. Similarly, although there is no momentous change at each tiny stage of development from zygote to person, still it is erroneous to say that an embryo is a person.

Second, the tiny size of the embryonic being whose entire existence is no larger than the period at the end of this sentence calls into question its moral significance. Just look at the embryo (if you can find it)! How can it possibly be equal in value to me!

Third, the fact that early embryos can twin forming two separate embryos leading to the birth of monozygotic "identical" twins casts doubt on whether there is an *individual* human present from conception. How can we say that an individual human life begins at conception if suddenly this "individual" human being becomes two individuals?

Fourth, two embryos conceived from two separate fertilized eggs can fuse together to become a single zygote. This fusion, like twining, calls into question whether such embryos really were individuals at all. These third and fourth arguments lead many to hold the "primitive streak" after which twinning and fusion is impossible, which marks the true beginning of an *individual* human life about two weeks after conception.

Fifth, scientists have estimated that more than 50% of zygotes spontaneously abort prior to live birth. Such a high rate of "wastage" casts doubt on the importance of the zygote and calls into question the authenticity of those who claim to believe life begins at conception, since such people rarely act to stop what they should believe is a massive loss of human life.

Sixth, some adopt an Aristotelian hylomorphic theory via Thomas Aquinas that a human being is made up of body and soul, and in order for a human soul to exist the human body must be proportioned to the rational soul. The body can only have a rational soul much later in pregnancy when rudimentary biological bases for rationality develop, so early in pregnancy the human embryo or fetus is not human.

Seventh, critics argue that the anti-abortion position entails the wrongfulness of some or all forms of contraception.

Eighth, the pro-life position implies the absurd view that every single cell of the human body has "a right to life," since every human cell has the potential to develop into a person like you or me via reproductive cloning.

Ninth, if forced to choose between rescuing ten frozen embryos or five adult patients, virtually everyone would choose the adults, so embryos must not be persons.

Tenth, the human embryo is not a human organism, since in the initial stages of development the individual cells that make up the embryo are more akin to a bag of marbles than coordinating parts of a unified organism.

Finally, some suggest that we ought to establish the boundaries of human personhood by means of a cost-benefit analysis of drawing the line in various places. When this analysis is undertaken, one has a strong argument against the embryo being a human person since both women, in the case of abortion, and other human beings, in the case of medical research using human embryos, could be greatly served by classifying human beings prior to birth as non-persons. Let us explore each argument in greater depth.

6.1 The Acorn Analogy

The first objection to embryonic personhood admits that an exact cut-off point between human non-persons and human persons may be difficult or even impossible to determine. For example, Judith Jarvis Thomson, whose work we will focus on in chapter seven, holds that the continuous development from the embryonic stage of development through more mature stages does not show that a person is present from conception. A human zygote is no more a person than an acorn is a full-grown tree (Thomson 1971, p. 48; Harris & Holm 2003, p. 119). Rosalind Hursthouse makes use of a different analogy to make the same point. Imagine a green patch left in the direct sun day after day, which over a long time fades to blue. There is no exact moment when the green patch turns to blue, but it is fallacious to argue that the patch must have really been blue all along. Similarly, the human being gradually becomes the person that is the healthy adult person. There is no "magic moment" of personhood, but we need not assume from the lack of such moment, that the human being from the very beginning of life is a person (Hursthouse 1987, pp. 36–38; Rubenfeld 1991, p. 625; Coleman 2004, p. 89).

How might one committed to the equality of all human beings respond to the acorn analogy and versions of it? There are at least two ways of taking the analogy about the acorn. The first is the supposition that the transition from acorn to oak tree involves a substantial change, the second that it does not. If we suppose that the transition involves a substantial change, that the acorn is one kind of thing and the oak tree is another kind of thing, then upon further reflection it becomes clear that the analogy is faulty in a number of ways. First, unlike a dormant and passive acorn, (again supposing this understanding of an acorn is correct), a human embryo is an active, self-developing organism (not a part of an organism) growing towards full maturity. Precisely at issue is whether the human embryo is the same kind of thing, substantially and ethically, as a human being at later developments of life, so we cannot appeal to the acorn analogy without begging this question.

Suppose, by contrast, that "acorn" is a phase in the development of one organism which moves through its lifespan from inception as an acorn into sapling into the full maturity of being an oak tree. Suppose, in other words, that the transition from acorn to oak tree involves no substantial change, but merely growth and development of the very same thing. If by "person" is meant "mature members of the human species," then of course, no human embryo is a person in this idiosyncratic sense of the term, but then again neither is any toddler. The proper analogy is therefore: Acorn is to oak tree as embryo is to *adult*. Obviously there are developmental differences between more and less maturely developed organisms be they plants, animals, or humans. Respecting human life from its inception does not commit one to the idea that all human beings are equally developed, that acorns are oak trees, or that embryos are adults. The difference between the two in each pair is maturity, but differences in maturity are not significant to personhood. The human toddler is immature, but no less a person than an adult.

Turning to another version of the same objection, it is true that no non-arbitrary line separates the green fading patch from the blue, and it is also true that the green patch was not really blue all along. But precisely at issue is whether the human being from the beginning of his or her life is a person, so to simply assert by analogy a negative answer (as green is not blue, so too the human embryo is not a person) is plainly to beg the question. A non-question begging and proper analogy (as green is not blue, so a very young human being is not an adult human being) does not serve, considered by itself, to justify the exclusive view that not all human beings are persons.

Imagine the debate is not (or is?) about infanticide rather than abortion. Critics of infanticide point out that none of the many differences between an adult and a newborn are morally significant in determining the right to life. There are many stages of development between infancy and adulthood, but these are not relevant to personhood. The defender of infanticide hardly establishes that a newborn baby is not a person by arguing from the following premises: (1) the process of development from infancy to adulthood admits no non-arbitrary moment when personhood is realized, and (2) the newborn baby is not an adult person. Both these premises are true, but the conclusion that a baby lacks a right to life does not follow. The baby is not an *adult* person, but its immaturity does not of itself show that a baby has no right to life.

Finally, as George and Lee note, the acorn analogy works only if one:

> disregards the key proposition asserted by opponents of embryo-killing: that all human beings, irrespective of age, size, stage of development, or condition of dependency, possess equal and intrinsic dignity by virtue of *what* (i.e., *the kind* of entity) they are, not in virtue of any accidental characteristics, which can come and go, and which are present in human beings in varying degrees. Oak trees and acorns are not equally valuable, because the basis for their value is not *what* they are but precisely those accidental characteristics by which oak trees differ from acorns. We value the ugly, decaying oak tree less than the magnificent, still flourishing one; and we value the mature, magnificent oak more than the small, still growing one. But we would never say the same about human beings.
>
> (2005, pp. 92–93)

Unlike acorns and oak trees, human value depends upon endowment rather than performance. So although it is foolish to say that destroying an acorn is no different than destroying an oak tree, the same is not true of destroying an embryo and destroying a more developed human. As Lee and George note, this is made more clear by the intuition that destroying a 100-year-old oak is worse than destroying a mere oak sapling (by virtue of the greater majesty and maturity of the oak), but killing a mature human being and a toddler are equal violations of the right to life despite their differences in age, maturity, intelligence, and other performative abilities (by virtue of their equal human dignity).

6.2 Size

How small is too small? The size of the human embryo or zygote has also called into question its humanity and/or its moral value. Can anyone honestly believe that just a few cells are a human being? Can anything that small be of any great significance? Just look at how different a zygote is from an adult human being? A prenatal human being in the third trimester of pregnancy may be a person, but a tiny human embryo smaller than a period certainly is not.

How could the pro-life advocate respond to such a critique? From a biological perspective, the size of a being plays no role in determining which species a being belongs to. Certainly, a newborn is smaller than a 10-year-old who in turn is smaller than an adult. But each of these are truly persons and undoubtedly human. We do not claim giant persons are more human so it is difficult to see why size would be decisive when considering small, even extremely small beings. Nor does size play a decisive role in determining personhood or the wrongfulness of killing. If size is what makes one a person, then we are faced again with the equality problem since various human persons differ in size. Indeed, to kill a child is often thought of as *worse* than killing an adult for a child is small and defenseless while most adults are not. Many things much smaller than a period, indeed entities so small as to be invisible to the naked eye entirely have incredible human significance, such as the HIV virus or penicillin. The human genome possessed by each human zygote, though tiny, consists of thirty-nine thousand genes, made up of 3.2 billion base pair sequences that, in terms of information directing the growth and development of a human being, has been compared to 200 New York City phone books (Cioffi 2001, p. 132).

Dean Stretton develops a variation on the normal argument from size by asking us to imagine a species called "shrinkers" that begin as embryos then develop through various stages of development towards maturity as rational adults. After a few years in this stage, they begin to shrink and regress all the way through the developmental stages to the zygotic stage, where they can remain alive as zygotes for five years. There is no way for shrinkers to attain functional rationality again. Stretton holds that we do nothing wrong by cutting their lifespan short. Since shrinkers do not have a right to live in virtue of having a natural capacity for rationality, neither do human embryos have a right to live in virtue of having a natural capacity for rationality (2008, p. 795).

As noted, size itself is completely irrelevant to personhood. If healthy adult human beings were somehow shrunk to tiny size, no one would deny their right to live. So let us posit a slightly different case of shrinkers to focus our intuitions on morally relevant characteristics. Imagine beings that do not shrink but remain basically the same size in maturity. However, like shrinkers, these beings who were once rational will never rationally function again. They have permanently lost their rational faculties. Indeed, we do not need to imagine such beings because they already exist. Severely mentally handicapped human beings fit the bill, at least those who became handicapped as adults. Advanced Alzheimer's patients are in the same condition, as are human beings with severe senility. Since it is morally wrong to kill these human beings intentionally, so, too, would it be wrong to kill shrinkers, whether they shrank or not. Thus, shrinkers provide no basis for denying basic respect to the human embryo.

Perhaps the fact that the human embryo begins as a *single* cell suggests that there is no human person present. Human beings are organisms composed of many cells. So at least at the zygotic stage, since there is only one cell present, there must not be an organism, and if there is no organism, then there is no human organism. And if there is no human organism, then there is obviously no human person.

However, although it is true that some organisms have many cells, there is no reason to think that all organisms by definition must have many cells, rather than simply many parts. Indeed, scientists recognize hundreds of species of single-celled organisms, including amoeba, euglena, and bacteria. Organisms must have parts that coordinate and function together for the good of the whole, but nothing excludes an organism from consisting of a single cell.

Dean Stretton offers a different argument, "At the first cell division, the single-celled zygote fissions into two duplicate cells. But no substance can survive fission into duplicates, and so we cannot identify the single-celled zygote with the subsequent organism" (2008, p. 797). Surely, the human person is a substance, but if so, it cannot be identical with the single-celled zygote.

A questionable premise of Stretton's argument is that the single-celled zygote fissions into two duplicate, identical cells, as takes place with amoebae. The first cell division in the zygote gives rise to two cells, one of which will give rise to the embryo proper; the other of which will give rise to the trophoblast (George and Tollefsen 2008a, pp. 154–155). These different developmental paths may be due to differences already present in each cell rather than to external influences. It is also questionable whether this division is properly described as fission:

> The main reason is that when a zygote divides a very important item is retained. Both at the initial stage and at the resulting two-cell stage there is not only a complete, connected external boundary, but, more precisely, a membrane or a physical covering—the *zona pellucida*—surrounding the cells. This membrane does not divide or disappear. The division takes place *within* its boundaries. . . . [T]he division of an amoeba by fission is *not* an adequate analogue to the division of a one-cell zygote. Amoebas do not retain a common external boundary

or membrane after they divide, nor do they start to specialize into amoebas with different, yet coordinated functions.

(Damschen, Gomez-Lobo, & Schonecker 2006, pp. 169, 171)

The initial division of the zygote could be described as the first cell giving rise to another cell and, though diminished in size, surviving the production of this other cell. The change in the embryo is a case of growth, not fission.

6.3 Twinning

Does twinning show that the human embryo at conception is not an individual human being? Many have asserted that it does (Warnock 2004, pp. 65–66). That depends on one's answer to a related question. Does the lack of the potentiality to give rise to a twin mark the beginning of an individual human life? The answer must be "no," since any adult human being can in principle be cloned. Cloning is simply an artificial form of twinning which replicates the human genetic code of the donor in order to create a being that is genetically an identical twin. Put another way, cloning makes it true that *every* being of human origin, from 24 hours after conception to 24 years after conception, can potentially give rise to a genetically identical human being. So the individuality of a human being must not arise from the lack of potential to twin.

A critic could reply that this response overlooks the difference between active and passive potentiality. The 24-year-old human has only passive potentiality to give rise to a cloned human being; whereas the 24-hour-old human has active potentiality to give rise to a twinned human being.

We do not know a great deal about how monozygotic twinning takes place, but it very well may be that the zygote has a merely passive potentiality to twin which is activated by forces outside the embryo. But even if the zygote had active potentiality to twin, it is hard to see why this property should count against the embryo being an individual, since active potentialities are properties enjoyed by individuals.

In any case, twinning does not show that there is no individual human being following conception. *Individuation*, being an individual, does not require *indivisibility* (Lee 1996, p. 93). The fact that one being can be divided into two beings does not mean that it was never an individual being. Most plants, for example, have totipotent cells that can give rise to further individual plants, but that does not mean that a plant cannot be an individual, distinct plant (Liao 2010b). Alfonso Gómez-Lobo provides another example that there is no necessary link between *indivisibility* and *individuality* noting that,

If indivisibility were a necessary condition for individuality, then there would be no material individuals. After all, any material object can be pulled apart or dismantled. No car would be an individual car, but only a collection or package of car parts, likewise no living body would be an individual organism, but only a colony of cells.

(2007, p. 458)

To use an organic example, if I cut a flatworm in half and it survives as two flatworms, it does not follow that the flatworm was really two flatworms all along or that the flatworm was never one individual worm.

Recognizing that the phenomena of twinning does not undermine the viewing conception as the beginning of a unique individual human being (individuality does not require indivisibility), McMahan offers a different reason based on twinning for thinking that a human zygote cannot be the beginning of a new human life:

> the embryo is someone like you or me and if it matters in the way you and I do (the two assumptions), then when symmetrical twinning occurs and an embryo ceases to exist, this should be tragic. For it is the ceasing to exist of someone who matters. According to the two assumptions, therefore, there is a serious moral reason to try to prevent monozygotic twinning from occurring. Or at least we should try to ensure that all instances of twinning involve asymmetrical division, so that no one ceases to exist. But these suggestions are absurd, and I know of no one who believes either.
>
> (2007, p. 178; Stretton 2008, p. 795)

But, why should we hold that the original twin has gone out of existence rather than that one twin has arisen from the original?

> [W]hen an embryo divides to form twins, if the division is symmetrical, the original embryo also ceases to exist. The original embryo cannot be identical with both twins, since one thing cannot be numerically identical with two things that are not identical with each other. And if the division is symmetrical, the original embryo cannot be one twin but not the other, for there is nothing about one twin to identify it as the original embryo that is not also true of the other.
>
> (McMahan 2007, p. 177)

McMahan moves from epistemological ignorance to metaphysical certainty. If we cannot know which of the two twins (if either) is the original, then we are not justified in concluding that the original has died. If we have no way of knowing which twin is the original, then one of them may very well be the original. Perhaps, McMahan should be understood as claiming that if the division is symmetric, there is nothing in virtue of which one twin could be said to be the original as opposed to the other twin.

This claim can be understood in at least two ways. Is the claim that by definition if the division is symmetrical, then by definition there could be nothing to identify one twin as the original as opposed to the other? If so, then this merely verbal point may be answered by the empirical question, is there really such a thing as symmetrical twinning? If the claim is not definitional, then symmetrical twinning could be such that something distinguishes one twin from the other so that one is the original but not the other. It very well could be that this differentiating characteristic has not yet been found, but will be found tomorrow. It could also be that there is no differentiating characteristic, so no such characteristic can ever be found. We simply do not know which is true at this point. As Stephen Napier points out, it is consistent with the empirical evidence to interpret twinning as a form of asexual reproduction in which the original zygote gives rise to another without every falling out of existence (Napier 2008). In other words, twinning may be a form of natural cloning or "budding" in which the original survives giving rise to another human being.

Even if we could know that the original zygote had ceased to exist in giving rise to the twins, it would still not follow that we would have a moral duty to combat twinning. Intervention in any given case of possible twinning would be virtually impossible in natural conception, since couples normally do not know if or when they conceive, let alone that they may be conceiving a zygote who will later become identical twins. Further, the burdens and benefits of treatment for all involved must also be taken into account in considering whether a given treatment is morally required to undertake or to continue. In this case, the burdens would likely be considerable. Indeed, it is a benefit to the twins that arise that the treatment *not* be provided. Even in cases where personhood is indisputably established, it is unreasonable in some cases to provide life-saving treatment. It is not a tragedy or a moral failure to fail to provide a heart transplant to a 95-year-old woman, even though she is uncontroversially a person.

6.4 Embryo Fusion

The other side of the twinning coin is *embryo fusion*. Just as an early embryo can split into two, so also two or more human embryos can fuse into one. The pro-choice argument is that two human beings cannot fuse into one, and since two embryos can fuse into one, human embryos must not be human individuals (Harris 1999, p. 296; Green 2001, p. 31). Rather, human embryos become "hominized" with the arrival of the primitive streak and the lack of the ability to fuse.

Unlike the case of embryo division and adult cloning, we have no examples of adult human beings who actually fuse into one. Of course, we didn't have cloning until the twenty-first century either, so the real question is whether being an individual human being *logically* implies that one cannot fuse with another human being. If something is logically possible, we may not be able to do it now, but it may well be possible to do it later as technology advances. Is it logically possible for two adult human beings to fuse into one? Or does the individuality of each human being logically exclude the fusion of two human beings? Fusing doesn't mean merely being joined together in fairly superficial ways, like Dante portrayed Paolo and Francesca in the second ring of the *Inferno* locked in perpetual sexual intercourse. There are cases of humans fusing depicted fairly recently which imagine the fusion in some sense of two human beings in various ways. In the movie *All of Me*, the character played by Lily Tomlin dies and through an accident ends up within the body of the character played by Steve Martin. The male and female psyches exist simultaneously and fight for dominance in Steve Martin's body (to great comic effect) until eventually Lily Tomlin's personality leaves. Or consider the *Star Trek* transporter that can break down the molecular structure of a human being in one place and then reassemble the person in a new place. In one episode, a transporter malfunctions turning two characters Tuvok and Neelix into a new combination, "Tuvix," a being not identical to either. Finally, if the father had eaten his children along with the breakfast cereal in *Honey I Shrunk the Kids*, the children would have been fused into him through the digestive process and would have ceased to exist as human beings and become one with his body.

Now how one analyzes these three cases Martin, *Star Trek*, and *Shrunk*, and whether they are all properly called fusions, will depend in part on what one believes about the relationship of body and soul, matter and spirit, or personality and corporality. The same is true for how one analyzes cases of embryo fusion (and twinning). Perhaps, two psyches can use one body, temporarily or permanently. Perhaps, two human beings cease to exist and a third comes into existence from the materials of the first two. Perhaps, one human being dies and nourishes the other who survives. Whatever one's view of the "mind/body problem" and how to understand the identity of the being arising from these cases of fusion, one thing is clear: in all three examples *two persons were present* before fusion. Martin, *Star Trek*, and *Shrunk* all show that the fusion of two into one does not in any way logically imply that there were not really two independent human beings prior to fusion. Since adult human beings could fuse with one another without logical contradiction, and no one doubts their humanity or personhood, it follows that human personhood is completely unrelated to the potentiality to fuse.

6.5 High Embryo-Mortality Rate

We simply do not know with precision the exact rate of early miscarriage. Some estimate it may be higher than 50%; others claim the actual rate is about 14% for healthy women (Grey & Wu 2000). Let's assume that the miscarriage rate is above 50%. Would this high percentage cast doubt on the human personhood of the early embryo? Not really. For centuries throughout the world, indeed until the twentieth century, the rate of infant mortality was more than 50%. In some places in Africa today, more than 50% of young people have died or will soon die from AIDS. A person might live only a day and a thing like a tree might live a century, but that doesn't make the tree a person or the person a thing. Death rates have no relationship to personhood.

Still, a problem remains. If people really believe that human life begins at completed conception, then they should mount a massive campaign to prevent these spontaneous miscarriages (Green 2001, p. 45; McMahan 2008, p. 188). Those that defend the value of human life from conception in cases of abortion and embryonic research do not show similar concern about other cases of loss of embryonic human life in spontaneous miscarriage.

However, as Green himself notes, miscarriages at any stage of pregnancy are, for a great many women as well as other family members, extremely traumatic experiences, more traumatic than simply not getting pregnant. Green's effort to de-emphasize the importance of the human embryo here overmasters his legitimate recognition that for many people the loss of a human embryonic or fetal life brings a time of great sadness and mourning.

But sadness or lack of sadness at a death is really beside the point when addressing whether a being is human or a person. The death of a lonely 90-year-old from a long bout with cancer may not cause sadness to anyone, but such a human being was surely as much a person as John F. Kennedy whose death caused intense mourning. We might weep bitterly over Old Yeller's death and be indifferent to old lady Haversham's death, but he's not a human person and she nevertheless is. Differences in emotional reactions to the news of a being's death hinge on many factors, including some obviously irrelevant to determining personhood—such as the beauty or celebrity of the deceased, how well we personally knew them, their achievements, and so forth.

The relatively high rate of "embryo loss," experts believe, results from grave abnormalities and serious deficiencies in the reproductive process, from incomplete fertilization. Thus, in perhaps the majority of cases a human being has not been formed and so a human being does not die, since conception itself has failed to be completed. However, given some percentage of loss of actual human embryos, could such losses be prevented? It is possible that efforts could be made with microsurgery or some other kind of intervention might save human embryos that would spontaneously miscarry, but almost certainly at great expense and burden to all those involved and with little hope of success.

However, not attempting to save embryonic life in this context simply does not indicate a tacit recognition that such human beings are not persons, or much less that they are not biologically human. Just as we often don't make extraordinary efforts to attempt to restore health to human beings in advanced old age, so we don't make extraordinary efforts to attempt to restore health to embryonic human beings. Neither implies a tacit recognition that the aged or embryonic are not fully persons or not fully human. An affirmation of the dignity of all human life simply does not imply that one must always make every effort to save human life regardless of the burdens involved or the likelihood of success. Even though every human life has intrinsic value, it does not follow that every proposed treatment is worthwhile or valuable regardless of promised benefits and likely burdens.

In addition, and unlike the case of the elderly dying, we really don't know with exact certainty the frequencies of early miscarriage. Even if we did know in general that early miscarriages happen fairly often, since we don't have windows to the womb, we generally have no knowledge that *this* woman bearing *this* human being within her is having a miscarriage *right now*. We are normally more concerned about the death of a well-known neighbor than the death of an unknown person thousands of miles away, so embryonic death at an early stage is generally less alarming than the death of a prenatal human being later in pregnancy.

If we did know exactly who was having a miscarriage, and if we had effective and non-burdensome ways to save this life, then the inclusive view would entail that we would have an obligation to try to save the human being in utero, and indeed a great many people would vigorously try—including the many people who suffer from infertility problems.

Martha Nussbaum offers another objection:

> First of all, it would appear that nobody consistently regards the fertilized ovum as a full-fledged person. Although this theological doctrine is paid lip service, people's practices suggest that it is not strictly interpreted. No religion holds funerals when there is a miscarriage. Women's menses are not inspected to see whether they contain a fertilized egg that has failed to implant. These facts suggest that even strict Roman Catholics do not really think that a person has died in such cases, or at least that they hold this in a half-hearted and not fully consistent way.
>
> (2008, p. 342)

Of course, generally we do not know if and when an embryo, or to use Nussbaum's dehumanizing term "fertilized egg," has died in utero, so it is not inconsistency but rather ignorance that prevents due acknowledgement of the loss of human life, a lack of knowledge that would likely not be remedied by inspecting women's menses.

Nussbaum's assertion, "No religion holds funerals when there is a miscarriage" is false. The Catholic Church teaches that "The corpses of human embryos and fetuses, whether they have been deliberately aborted or not, must be respected just as the remains of other human beings" (Congregation for the Doctrine of the Faith [CDF] 1987, section I, 4), so miscarried babies can and do receive Catholic funerals. Likewise, Protestant churches have conduced funeral services following both miscarriage and abortion. In Islam, funeral prayers should be said for the fetus if death occurs after ensoulment (Fataawa al-Lajnah al-Daa'imah, 21/434–438). In Buddhism, the *mizuko kuyo* is a memorial service performed for the deceased fetus. In Hinduism, the unborn are depicted as having great value from the very beginning of their lives (immediate hominization), having abilities similar to mature human persons such as hearing, learning, and remembering in utero (Bhattacharyya 2006, 86); and in the case of premature death, prayers are offered for their departed souls. Orthodox Judaism is an exception that proves too much, for in this tradition no funeral is required unless the baby survives 30 days *after birth*. So unless Nussbaum is willing to deny moral status to newborn babies in the first month of life, appeal to this Jewish practice will not be of much help in denying the moral status of unborn human life.

Even if Nussbaum were correct that no religion offered funerals following miscarriage, it would still not follow that this lack indicates a tacit denial of the moral status of the human beings prior to birth. If one understood funerals as services for the sake of the living, to comfort and console them in their loss rather than as services owed to the dead for their own sake, in cases where little or no loss is experienced by the living, as is the case where the deceased human being was not known well, there would be no need for a funeral. As mentioned earlier, the fact that the death of a human being is not experienced as a loss or cause for sadness by other human beings does not change the moral status that the deceased human being had.

6.6 Hylomorphism

According to this view, originating in Aristotle and defended by Thomas Aquinas as well as by some contemporary proponents (Donceel 1970; Ford 1988; McCormick 1991), the human embryo cannot have a soul until the body of the embryo, the "matter," is proportioned to receive a rational soul, the "form." As Donceel first put the argument:

> The main philosophical principles are as follows. The soul is the substantial form of man. A substantial form can exist only in matter

capable of receiving it. In the case of man's soul this means: the human soul can exist only in a highly organized body. . . . Yet, at the start there is not at once a highly organized body, a body with sense organs and a brain.

(1970, pp. 79, 80)

So until the embryo or fetus has a body sufficiently developed for rational functioning, the embryo or fetus is not "ensouled" and therefore not a human person.

Of course, the easiest way around this argument for those who oppose abortion or lethal research on human embryos is simply to deny the relevance of hylomorphic theory—the "soul" simply does not or should not come into the discussion of moral issues. Others have suggested that this argument proves too much—not only are embryos not human beings (let alone persons) but infants as well are not human beings since only three months after birth does an infant have the biological presupposition required for reflective mental activity (Lee 1996, p. 89). Even if one agrees with Tooley that newborns are not persons, it would be difficult, to say the least, to deny that babies are *biologically* human, members of *Homo sapiens*.

Even if one accepts some form of hylomorphism in which the human person is a unity of body and soul, an ensouled body, there is ample room for criticizing Aquinas's view as arising from a faulty understanding of the scientific facts. Thomas Aquinas certainly held a version of hylomorphism, but his belief that the embryo was not a human being did not arise so much from his understanding of Aristotle as from his ignorance of basic biological processes. Thomas's views on early human development hopelessly have been surpassed by contemporary science. As Aquinas scholar Mark Johnson writes:

> As a committed student of Thomas's writings, I must confess that none of his efforts on this issue [of human embryology and ensoulment] is salvageable. It is simply not possible to "tweak" what Thomas has said, for the very simple reason that the entire embryological basis upon which Thomas's argument rests, and from which the trajectory of his later claims about delayed hominization takes its origin, is factually false, and completely so. Thomas thought that the male's seed did not become one with the female's material contribution, which he believed was in such a crude state that effort was needed to bring the maternal contribution to even a minimal state of life; that is false, for we know now that the sperm and the egg prior to fertilization are highly and equally organized, though "half-organized," as it were, such that the union of the two at fertilization results in a single body that is materially one, and formally or organizationally one, and is indeed

organizationally more sophisticated than either the sperm or the egg had been, on its own, prior to fertilization — after fertilization occurs, of course, it is improper in the discipline of biology to speak further of "the sperm" or "the egg," since those two erstwhile realities no longer exist, but have become "parts" of another whole. Thomas thought that the embryo was the passive recipient of the semen's agency, since the semen worked-over, and shaped, and "built" the structures in the passive embryo, first developing in it the structures necessary for nutrition, then eventually sensation, and so on; that [too] is false.

(2002, p. 196)

So if one rejects the outdated biology, but accepts some version of hylomorphism in which human persons are embodied spirits or ensouled bodies, what should be said about the human embryo? Put another way, if Thomas were familiar with modern embryology and retained his philosophical beliefs, what would he hold about the beginning of human existence? Benedict Ashley and Albert Moraczewski answer:

The principle organ required by [Thomas's] argument need not be one that here and now is capable of acting as the instrument of intellection. We are human persons even when we are asleep or comatose from a brain injury. Instead, for Aquinas a living organism is one capable of acting as the *proportionate efficient cause* of its own self-organization and other vital activities. Thus the primary organ that is required in the fetus for its intellectual ensoulment is not the brain as such but a primary organ capable of producing a brain with the capacity for intellectual cognition in the body at some appropriate phase of the human life cycle. What is the primary organ that causes the human body to develop so as to be proportionate to ensoulment and human personhood? Modern embryology shows clearly that it is the nucleus of the zygote produced by the fertilization of a human ovum by a human sperm, since that nucleus 1) contains all the genome or *information* (formal cause) required to build the mature human body with its brain as its primary organ and the instrument of intellection and 2) is the principal *efficient cause* proportionate to the task of mature development of the human organism.

(Ashley and Moraczewski 2001, pp. 199–200,
emphasis in the original)

In other words, if one applies the philosophical principles adduced by Thomas Aquinas to the findings of contemporary embryology, then one arrives at the personhood of the embryo (see too, Haldane and Lee, 2003).

6.7 Anti-Abortion, Anti-Contraception

Stephen Coleman argues that defending embryonic personhood leads to difficulties in drawing distinctions between abortion and some forms of contraception. He holds that since the Intra-Uterine Device (IUD) and the pill can cause early abortions, critics of abortion should condemn them just as strongly as they condemn later surgical abortions (Coleman 2004, p. 91). Although many people who oppose abortion also oppose contraception, not all do. Even those who oppose contraception do not hold it as morally on a par with abortion. Coleman sees this as inconsistent, at least for forms of contraception that sometimes act as abortifacients.

There are two important differences between these potentially abortifacient forms of contraception and a typical abortion, which in part explains the different attitude taken by critics of abortion to each. As will be explored in greater length in chapter eight, one may do an act that has two effects, one good and one evil, if the evil is not used as a means or as an end, and if there is a proportionately serious reason.

There is also a difference between opposing what *may* cause harm as a side effect and opposing what is *aimed at* causing harm. The forms of contraception discussed here may (or may not) perform as abortifacients, while other forms of abortion, such as the use of RU-486 or surgical abortions, intentionally aim at destruction of the embryo.

Thus, those who consistently oppose abortion need not oppose all uses of "emergency contraception." For example, the ethical directives of U.S. Roman Catholic bishops for Catholic health-care facilities indicate that:

> A female who has been raped should be able to defend herself against a potential conception from the sexual assault. If, after appropriate testing, there is no evidence that conception has occurred already, she may be treated with medications that would prevent ovulation, sperm capacitation, or fertilization.
> (United States Council of Catholic Bishops [USCCB] 2001)

An opposition to abortion does not entail an opposition to contraception in general, nor does opposition to abortion entail an exceptionless opposition to contraception that *sometimes* prohibits implantation. It is permissible to *risk* the well-being of others for a proportionately serious reason. This would seem to leave open the possibility of using medicines which are contraceptive and may risk impeding implantation in cases of rape.

There is no logical inconsistency in opposing all abortion but not opposing contraception, since contraception, as indicated by its very name, acts against conception of a new human being. Abortion, on the other hand, terminates the life of a new human being. As Don Marquis notes in defending his own argument against abortion:

> An individual now has that sort of future of value just in case a later phase of that same individual would have a future it would value at later times and it has a future like ours. Accordingly, that earlier phase of that individual and those later phases of that individual must be phases of the *same* individual. That a UFO [Un-Fertilized Ovum] does not meet this condition can be shown by the following argument. Suppose the UFO that was my precursor was the same individual as I. Since identity is transitive, it follows that the UFO was my precursor and the sperm that was my precursor were the same individual. This is false.
>
> (2007, p. 407)

The anti-abortion position does not entail, contra Monty Python, that every sperm is sacred.

6.8 Living Human Cells Are Not Persons

Since virtually each living cell of the human body is genetically complete, living, and human, the pro-life view would seem to entail that any kind of "killing" of human cells is not different than killing a human person (Rubenfeld 1991, pp. 621–626; Harris & Holm 2003, p. 120). Aside from gametes, all cells of the human body are genetically complete and could develop into embryos through cloning. Thus, to rest personhood on mere genetic completeness excludes not just abortion, not just contraception, but "killing" any human cell whatsoever.

Although it is true that virtually every cell of the human body is genetically complete, the possibility of cloning is not a difficulty for the view that personhood begins at conception. Cloning makes it possible that each cell of the human body can develop into a mature human being, a genetic twin of the cell donor. A human fetus, however, does not merit protection in terms of its *potential* to develop, but rather in virtue of what it already actually is. A human embryo in utero is already and actually a whole, self-developing member of the human species. In other words, the pro-life claim does not rest on the *potentiality* of the embryo but on its *actuality*. A human cell like a skin or liver cell is not a whole member of the human species, but a part of a whole member of the human species. Such human cells are not actually self-developing towards human maturity. If human cloning became a reality, virtually any human cell would have the *potential* to become what a human embryo *actually* is: a whole, self-integrated, and self-actualizing human being developing towards human maturity.

An egg or sperm, indeed any individual cell of a human being's body is, by contrast, not a distinct, whole member of the human species, but rather a part of a distinct, whole, living member. Sperm and eggs lack genetic completeness, lack distinctiveness, and cannot self-actualize and develop towards human maturity. Neither egg nor sperm is a whole human being; both are parts of human beings. Unlike sperm and eggs, and unlike living human cells that are simply parts of a human being's body, the human embryo is a distinct, whole, and complete organism actively self-developing towards maturity and rational functioning.

John Harris argues that conception cannot be the beginning of a new human life because "conception can result in a hydatidiform mole, a cancerous multiplication of cells that will never become anything but a palpable threat to the life of the mother" (1999, p. 295; Harris and Holm 2003, p. 118). However, a hydatidiform mole results not from conception but from a failed attempt at conception, and, as Harris rightly notes, such moles do not constitute a being with a right to life, despite being a mass of human tissue. Such molar pregnancies are not even properly speaking organisms, so they cannot be human beings (who will always be organisms of a particular species—*Homo sapiens*). As such then molar pregnancies constitute no problem for the view that (most) human beings arise at conception.

Dean Stretton provides another argument against the idea that the early human embryo is the same beings as the human fetus, let alone the human newborn.

> The vast majority of the cells in the very early embryo go towards the creation of the placenta and amniotic sac rather than the later embryo. Thus we cannot identify the very early embryo with the later embryo, because the very early embryo has a better claim to being identical with the placenta or amniotic sac.
>
> (2008, p. 797, citations omitted)

The false assumption of this argument is that the placenta and amniotic sac are not parts of the human being in question, but something other than the human embryo. However, both the placenta and amniotic sac are in fact organs of the developing human being. They share the genetic makeup of the embryonic human beings rather than the mother. The fact that these organs are shed at a later stage of development does not entail that they are not parts of the human being at an earlier stage of development. Some parts or developmental aspects of a human being, like baby teeth or secondary sex characteristics, are temporary organs that are truly parts of a human being, during certain phases of development, but can be lost (baby teeth) or gained (secondary sex characteristics) as the human organism moves through the various stages of development.

Even if the placenta and amniotic sac were not parts of the human being in question, it would still not follow that the very early embryo is identical with the placenta or amniotic sac. The very early embryo cannot be identical with the placenta, amniotic sac, or even the later human embryo because there are many important differences among them. Many things, most obviously size, are true of the early embryo but not true of the placenta or amniotic sac. If we construe "identical" as meaning "arising from," then the placenta, amniotic sac, and the later human embryo all are identical with the very early embryo.

6.9 Embryo Rescue Case

Dean Stretton imagines a case in which an emergency arises and a person is faced with the choice of rescuing ten frozen human embryos or five adult patients. Since virtually everyone would choose to save the adult patients rather than the embryos, this indicates that the patients have a higher moral status than the frozen human embryos (Stretton 2008, p. 795).

As noted earlier (section 4.3), we have moral justification for treating human beings enjoying basic equal human rights in different ways. If forced to choose between saving the President of the United States and four other national Presidents and Prime Ministers, rather than ten unknown patients, most people would choose the Presidents and the Prime Ministers. To choose to save Presidents and Prime Ministers rather than plain persons is not a denial of the equal basic rights of those not saved, but rather a recognition that deaths of world leaders adversely effects many more people than the deaths of regular patients. Similarly, in virtue of the fact that the adult patients have received an "investment" from their parents and society in terms of education and upbringing, have future plans that would be thwarted, have responsibilities to discharge, and have strong relationships with others, it makes sense to choose to save five adult persons rather than ten frozen embryos. In choices about who to save, various circumstances can determine who is chosen without a denial of the fundamental equality of the human beings involved. The embryo rescue case does not show that human embryos lack basic human rights (see also, Liao 2006a).

6.10 The Bag of Marbles Analogy

Human beings are organisms having various parts that contribute to the good of the whole. By contrast, a bag of marbles or a heap of shoes consists of various individual things in proximity to one another, but each of the things is a "free agent" without a role in an organized structure, unfettered to receiving and making contributions to the whole (Warnock 2004, p. 65). The cells of the early human embryo within the embryonic membrane the *zona pellucida* are akin to a bag of marbles rather than to an organism since the various cells are integrated and interactive with each other for the sake of the whole. Modifying the bag of marble argument, others admit some interaction between the cells but posit that the interaction is insufficient for the being to be considered an organism or that it is unclear whether or not the being is an organism (Stretton 2008, p. 797).

One difficulty with the bag of marbles analogy is there is evidence that the cells of the early human embryo are interacting with one another and becoming specialized so as to contribute to the development of a mature human body. S. Matthew Liao argues,

> there are thousands of cells by the time a blastula is formed around the nine-day stage, and certainly many more by the sixteen day stage. Though by no means metaphysically impossible, it seems highly suspect that these thousands of cells would all be distinct and separate organisms; that they would not be sufficiently coordinated; and that at the sixteen-day stage, all of them would all of a sudden become sufficiently coordinated to compose a single organism.
>
> (2010b, p. 64)

As Robert P. George and Christopher Tollefson argue in their book *Embryo: A Defense of Human Life*, the early human embryo acts so as to achieve certain goals including preventing more than one sperm from fertilizing the egg, moving into the uterus, making implantation possible, and overcoming various threats to its existence. In achieving these goals, the various cells of the embryo must work together, communicate to overcoming obstacles to achieving these goals, and develop further cells of greater specification. George and Tollefson cite the embryologist Bruce Carlson who notes:

> Even at the early stage the blastomeres of a cleaving embryo are not homogenous. Simple staining methods reveal pronounced differences among cells in human embryos as early as the seven-cell stage. Autoradiographic studies have shown that all blastomere of four-cell human embryos have low levels of extranucleolar and nonnucleolar RNA synthesis. By the eight-cell stage, some blastomeres have very high levels of RNA synthesis, but other blastomeres still show the pattern seen in blastomeres of the four-cell embryo. Morphological studies show corresponding differences between transcriptionally active and inactive blastomeres.
>
> (2008a, p. 154)

If the human embryo is not an organism, in virtue of what can this loose collection of cells accomplish these tasks?

In his article, "Killing Embryos for Stem Cell Research," Jeff McMahan admits that there is some unity and interaction between these cells, if only a unity and interaction needed to produce the more mature stages of human development, but perhaps there is insufficient unity and interaction for these cells to constitute an organism. After all, immediately following the death of a mature human being, there remains a high level of organization among the remaining living tissues of the corpse, and yet the newly dead corpse is not an organism (McMahan 2007, p. 180).

The reason that the newly dead corpse is not an organism, the reason why it is properly considered dead rather than alive despite various cells in the body continuing to live, is that its parts no longer function as integrated, coordinate parts of a whole, contributing and receiving in coordination with, so as to contribute to the health and functioning of the whole. As Maureen Condic notes,

> Embryos are in full possession of the very characteristic that distinguishes a living human being from a dead one: the ability of all cells in the body to function together as an organism, with all parts acting in an integrated manner for the continued life and health of the body as a whole.
>
> (2003, p. 52)

The human embryo has sufficient organization to develop towards greater maturity and function as a being of its kind. Since this level of organization is sufficient for being considered an "organism" at every other stage of development along the life span, sufficient for distinguishing living from dead organisms, it should be considered sufficient organization for being an organism also at the beginning of life.

Some people have noted that the embryo does indeed have directedness towards human maturity, but they object that the embryo lacks *inner* directedness characteristic of an organism. The embryo's developmental trajectory is governed by maternal RNA, not by the embryo's own genetic endowment. In the words of Stretton,

> Organisms during their early stages exhibit self-directed development, or in other words development "from within"; but the zygote's development until the four to eight cell stage is externally directed by the mother's RNA (inherited from the ovum), and so the zygote during this phase is not an organism.
>
> (2008, p. 797)

A similar charge is leveled by William Saletan in a *New York Times Book Review* of *Embryo: A Defense of Human Life* by Robert P. George and Christopher Tollefsen.

George and Tollefsen respond:

> The RNA is "maternal" only in the sense that it is contributed by the oocyte. But as human embryologist Maureen Condic explains,

"once an embryo has come into existence, the maternally derived RNA, like the embryo's genome, belong to the embryo itself. They are not components of the mother, somehow acting at a distance, but components of the embryo acting to further its own development." They form aspects of the complete developmental program of the embryo and are neither extrinsic, nor distinct agents. (Nor do they cause the embryo of some early stage to become a numerically different being.) These facts discredit Saletan's claim—central to his case against our position—that "maternal factors don't just facilitate the embryo's program; they direct it." The truth is that the embryo's development is internally directed. The embryo directs not only its own integral organic functioning, but also its development in the direction of maturity as a member of the human species.

(2008b)

No one denies that the early embryo, indeed the later embryo and human fetus is influenced by many maternal factors. Indeed, the influence goes both ways with the mother being influenced also by even the early embryo. Such two-way interactions continue after birth when newborns nurse. But none of these influences or interactions undermines the identity as a distinct organism of the mother and the offspring.

6.11 Cost–Benefit Analysis

Finally, some suggest that we should determine the beginning of personhood by means of judging the costs and benefits of "drawing the line" in various places (see Rubenfeld 1991, p. 600). However, if personhood depends upon the weighing of costs involved in granting personhood against the costs to others, the door is opened, in certain circumstances, for that calculus to lead to the denial of personhood even to rationally functioning adults, whether as individuals or as members of a class. Although this reasoning is often used to justify the death penalty, even the rights and dignity of the innocent could not be secured by this kind of justification. Green writes:

The alternative to abuse and exclusion is not to obscure the need for choice and decision in these matters, but to make choice explicit and to be prepared to rationally defend one's criteria before the entire human moral community. Every member of this community has a vital stake in these matters, and every person has a right to be aware of and to participate in these determinations.

(2001, p. 52)

However, one can hardly determine who is a member of the human moral community by discussion with members of the human moral community.

This circular reasoning undermines Green's justification of lethal human embryo research. Precisely the question at issue is who counts as "us" and "everyone" whose interests, potential or actual, weigh in the deliberation. By its nature, a cost–benefit analysis of whatever kind cannot determine *who* should benefit nor what counts as a *cost* or a *benefit* (MacIntyre 1992). So a cost–benefit analysis is incapable of answering questions of personhood.

6.12 The Uncertainty Argument

Now, many philosophers have noted that even if there is a reasonable probability that a human person is present from conception, we should not proceed with abortion. Imagine if a building were slated for demolition. Suddenly, a few persons arrive urging that the demolition not proceed because there were human beings still left inside. It would be gravely irresponsible to destroy the building in such circumstances until these concerns were adequately addressed. Or imagine a hunter who could not determine whether the movement behind the bush was caused by a wolf or by a person. The hunter has an obligation not to fire until determining that no person will be injured. Hence, if weighty questions remain about the personhood of the human embryo, it would be unjust to kill such a being precisely because serious doubts arise about the status of this being.

This consideration is immeasurably strengthened by recalling that in every other instance where personhood was denied to a class of human beings, we judge that a moral catastrophe took place. Since the human/person distinction has thus far had a 100% rate of failure, it is reasonable to adopt the inclusive view: every human being is a person.

Might one equally claim that, if there is any reasonable chance that fetuses are not persons (lack a right to life), we shouldn't drastically limit women's reproductive liberty? After all, the human fetus may not be a person, and this would surely impinge upon the reproductive liberty of women to consider abortion morally impermissible.

There is, however, an important difference between the two cases. To have one's reproductive liberty curtailed is a serious matter, but a much more serious matter is to have one's very life ended which also takes away any possibility for reproductive liberty. The degree of possible damage in the first case is very serious, but in the other case is absolutely catastrophic.

In addition, one could just as well say that, if there is any reasonable chance that newborn babies lack a right to life, we should not drastically limit women's and men's reproductive liberty to decide whether they will become parents to the person who will emerge later from the baby. As noted in chapter two, serious questions have been asked about the personhood of newborn babies, and it does indeed curtail the reproductive liberties of not just women but also men to forbid infanticide.

Does the uncertainty argument also entail that no one should eat meat? After all, if pigs and cows have a right to live, then serious wrongs are done in killing them for food. If pigs and cows do not have a right to live, then if we've given up meat, we've lost some enjoyment in eating but not risked violating another's rights.

The subject of animal rights is an interesting and important topic, but this book does not take any position on the matter either for or against. To be for or against abortion does not entail being for or against animal rights. Does the uncertainty argument entail that we ought not to eat meat? Not necessarily, for if one were quite certain that animals do not have rights, then the certainty argument would not apply. By contrast, since every previous time we have distinguished human persons from human non-persons we have made a moral mistake, I'm not sure how someone could claim to know with certainty that a certain class of human beings do not count as persons.

However, even if every human being is a person, abortion may still be morally permissible. After all, common intuition holds that it is not wrong to kill other people in, for example, self-defense and just war. Indeed, many defenders of abortion have seen the choice to terminate pregnancy as precisely a kind of defensive action. It is to these perspectives that we now turn.

7   Is it Wrong to Abort a Person?

If every human fetus is a person, is abortion always wrong? It would seem so. Since having others respect one's right to life is a *necessary condition* for the possibility of enjoying all other rights (including the right to privacy and bodily integrity), it has a necessary priority over all other rights (Spitzer 2000, pp. 240–242). To undermine someone's right to life is also to undermine all his or her other rights. As Martha Nussbaum notes about the right to abortion,

> The standard argument in favor of such a right has been an argument grounded in the notion of *privacy*. This argument is highly vulnerable to the metaphysical issue. If the fetus is a full-fledged person, then an appeal to privacy does not help us to defend abortion rights, just as privacy would not help us to justify infanticide, or child abuse.
>
> (2008, p. 342, emphasis in the original)

So, if the human fetus is a person, does this mean that abortion is always wrong?

"No," answers Judith Jarvis Thomson in an article entitled "A Defense of Abortion" originally published in 1971. Thomson's essay is the most famous article ever written about the subject of abortion, indeed one of the most frequently reprinted articles in twentieth century philosophy. In this article, Thomson offers a number of considerations that would justify abortion in the vast majority of cases without denying the personhood of the human fetus. Even if human personhood begins at the conception of a new human being, nevertheless, according to Thomson, abortion is (normally) permissible.

7.1 The Violinist Analogy

Thomson uses a series of analogies to defend this conclusion, the most famous of which is the violinist analogy. Imagine the following scenario:

> You wake up in the morning and find yourself back to back in bed with an unconscious violinist. A famous unconscious violinist. He has been found to have a fatal kidney ailment, and the Society of Music Lovers has canvassed all the available medical records and found that you alone have the right type of blood to help. They have therefore kidnapped you, and last night the violinist's circulatory system was plugged into yours, so that your kidneys can be used to extract poisons from his blood as well as your own. The director of the hospital now tells you, "Look, we're sorry the Society of Music Lovers did this to you—we would never have permitted it if we had known. But still, they did it, and the violinist now is plugged into you. To unplug you would be to kill him. But never mind, it's only for nine months. By then he will have recovered from his ailment, and can safely be unplugged from you." Is it morally incumbent on you to accede to this situation? No doubt it would be very nice of you if you did, a great kindness. But do you *have* to accede to it? What if it were not nine months, but nine years? Or longer still? What if the director of the hospital says, "Tough luck, I agree, but now you've got to stay in bed, with the violinist plugged into you, for the rest of your life." Because remember this. All persons have a right to life, and violinists are persons. Granted you have a right to decide what happens in and to your body, but a person's right to life outweighs your right to decide what happens in and to your body. So you cannot ever be unplugged from him.
>
> (Thomson 1971, p. 48–49)

But were you to find yourself in such a situation, would you really be morally required to remain attached to the violinist? Thomson thinks not. One can unplug oneself from the violinist without doing something that is morally impermissible. So abortion, the "unplugging" from oneself of the human fetus, is not necessarily unjust, *even if* the human being in utero is, like the violinist, fully a person. In other words, the human fetus may have a right to life, but this right to life does not include the right to make use of a woman's body. A woman has the right to disconnect herself from the human fetus, and this does not violate the fetus's right to life, even if such disconnection ends the fetus's life.

Now a "Good Samaritan," says Thomson, might go out of his way to save the life of the violinist. In clarifying what is meant by a Good Samaritan, Thomson quotes from the Gospel of Luke (10:30–35) in which Jesus describes the proverbial Good Samaritan as having cared for a person who had fallen among thieves. A Good Samaritan is someone who goes above and beyond the call of duty, executing not just obligatory but also supererogatory acts. But such heroic action is clearly not required for an agent to be minimally decent and avoid wrongdoing. It would be wonderful if everyone gave 50% of his or her income to the poor or spent each weekend serving the needs of the homeless at local soup kitchens. However, not to perform such generous acts does not make a person vicious. A person who is not a Good Samaritan is not necessarily evil, even if he or she doesn't merit our admiration either.

Therefore, one may refuse to undertake such heroic service and nevertheless remain what Thomson calls a "Minimally Decent Samaritan." Although the Minimally Decent Samaritan could stay plugged into the violinist, it does not follow that he is a wrongdoer if he does not. A Good Samaritan may have remained attached, but unplugging oneself from the human being in utero is entirely compatible with being a Minimally Decent Samaritan, who at least does not shirk any moral duty, even though, unlike the Good Samaritan, he does not go *above and beyond* the call of duty. Although heroic action was not undertaken, no moral wrongdoing took place.

Even if the human fetus has a right to life, the human being in utero doesn't have a right to use his or her mother's body, and this use, if granted, is a heroic act on the part of the mother. It is, in other words, the act of a Good Samaritan.

One objection to the violinist analogy considered by Thomson in her original article is that waking up finding yourself hooked up to the violinist is like waking up pregnant from a rape, but not like most cases of pregnancy where both the man and woman have voluntarily done an act that has led to the conception of human life. Since cases of rape make up only about 1% of all abortions, Thomson's violinist analogy would cover only a small percentage of cases. To make the cases more closely analogous, imagine that attending certain concerts brought with it (as a natural, though perhaps not intended, consequence) the possibility of getting hooked up to a violinist. Indeed, suppose that attending a concert was sometimes also called "getting hooked up to a violinist," as sexual acts are also known as reproductive acts. In the vast majority of cases, the woman and the man who brought about the pregnancy, knowingly and willingly performed an action with their reproductive organs that they realized could result in a pregnancy. Indeed, they consented to an action that is biologically ordered to reproduction, and therefore very much unlike a person who just "wakes up" hooked up to the violinist. In responding to objection such as these, Thomson supplies another analogy to illustrate that a woman may disconnect herself from the human fetus.

7.2 The Burglar Analogy

Taking into account the objection that the violinist analogy only covers cases of pregnancy through rape, Thomson suggests another analogy to indicate why abortion is justifiable even if the fetal-human person is not conceived as a result of rape.

If the room is stuffy, and I therefore open a window to air it, and a burglar climbs in, it would be absurd to say, "Ah, now he can stay, she's given him a right to the use of her house—for she is partially responsible for his presence there, having voluntarily done what enabled him to get in, in full knowledge that there are such things as burglars, and that burglars burgle." It would be still more absurd to say this if I had had bars installed outside my windows, precisely to prevent burglars from getting in, and a burglar got in only because of a defect in the bars.

(Thomson 1971, p. 58–59)

In this analogy, the human fetus is like a burglar breaking into a house with an open window. If someone were to trespass through a window left ajar, it may be praiseworthy to exercise tremendous patience and to wait for the burglar to leave, but there is no blame in expelling such an unwanted guest from your house, even if the person would die as a result. In the same way, a woman can remove an unwanted human person from within her body. Expulsion of a burglar would be even more justified if bars had been placed over the windows and doors, and the burglar got in anyway. In like manner, those who use contraception but conceive anyway have special warrant for expelling the human fetus. In general, there is greater justification for removing an intruder (be it burglar or human fetus) from where he or she shouldn't be (one's home or womb), even if such removal must be by death-dealing force, when one has taken extra steps in attempting to ensure that no one unwanted enters. In her book, *Breaking the Abortion Deadlock: From Choice to Consent*, Eileen McDonagh argues in a similar way, holding that the human fetus must be held accountable for what it does, for the fetus "imposes the serious injuries of wrongful pregnancy even if the pregnancy is medically normal" (McDonagh 1996, p. 7). Thus a human being in utero should be treated as an aggressor who may be repelled with lethal force.

Following on the burglar analogy, Thomson suggests a third analogy to show that even if the human fetus were fully a person, abortion would still be permissible.

Again, suppose it were like this: people-seeds drift about in the air like pollen, and if you open your windows, one may drift in and take root in your carpets or upholstery. You don't want children, so you fix up your windows with fine mesh screens, the very best you can buy. As can happen, however, and on very, very rare occasions does happen, one of the screens is defective; and a seed drifts in and takes root. Does the person-plant who now develops have a right to the use of your house? Surely not—despite the fact that you voluntarily open your windows, you knowingly kept carpets and upholstered furniture, and you knew that screens were sometimes defective.

Someone may argue that you are responsible for its rooting, that it does have a right to your house, because after all you could have lived out your life with bare floors and furniture, or with sealed windows and doors. But this won't do—for by the same token anyone can avoid a pregnancy due to rape by having a hysterectomy, or anyway by never leaving home without a (reliable!) army.

(Thomson 1971, p. 59)

So, on one side of the debate, the fact that the human fetus is not consciously and deliberately trying to trespass is not important in determining whether the human fetus has the right to be supported by the mother. Without being invited in, trespassers, whether guilty or innocent, may be forcefully expelled from house or uterus since they do not have the right to make use of house or uterus.

Having given three analogies in defense of abortion, Thomson foresees another line of argumentation against all these analogies, namely that parents have a special kind of responsibility for their own children that strangers do not have to anonymous violinists, burglars, or floating people-plants (Thomson 1971, p. 65). To be a minimally decent parent one must do many things that if done to strangers would make a person a Good Samaritan, indeed a Splendid Samaritan, a heroically good person. To clothe, feed, house, and look after the education of someone for 18 years (indeed characteristically longer) is what is minimally expected of a decent parent, but obviously would be a supererogatory or heroic action if undertaken for a stranger.

However, Thomson denies that special duties arise from the biological parent–child relationship. A pregnant woman does not have duties to the human fetus, says Thomson.

Surely we do not have any such "special responsibility" for a person unless we have assumed it, explicitly or implicitly. If a set of parents do not try to prevent pregnancy, do not obtain an abortion, and then at the time of birth of the child do not put it out for adoption, but rather take it home with them, then they have assumed responsibility for it, they have given it rights, and they cannot now withdraw support from it at the cost of its life because they find it difficult to go on providing for it. But if they have taken all reasonable precautions against having a child, they do not simply by virtue of their biological relationship . . . have a special responsibility for it.

(Thomson 1971, p. 65)

A key facet of the argument is the claim that special responsibilities only exist if explicitly or implicitly assumed, and that in most cases the pregnant woman has not assumed this special responsibility for the human fetus within her. Therefore, she has no obligation to allow this person to remain "plugged in," though if she wishes to be a Good Samaritan she may of course do so.

7.3 The "No Worse Off" Argument

Francis Kamm develops another way of justifying abortion even if the human fetus is a person. Her complex and detailed argument hinges on the following claim:

> By being killed and harmed in order to end a pregnancy, a fetus loses only the life that is provided by the woman's support, support which is not required by its need and any special obligation; it is not harmed relative to prospects it had before its attachment to the woman's body (and it is not worse off than it would have been if it had never been in the woman's body); and killing the fetus does not cause it to lose anything that the woman is causally responsible for its having that it would retain independently of her. That is, the fetus had no opportunities before being attached to the woman's body (i.e., before its conception) of which it would be deprived, and it would have had no opportunities other than being attached to the woman's body. It is also no worse off being dead because it was killed than if it had never existed.
>
> (Kamm 1992, p. 80, emphasis removed)

Kamm's argument presupposes something that was also argued for by Thomson, namely that the mother has no duty to provide aid for her fetus. Given that there is no such duty, and given that the fetus is no worse off being killed than never having existed, abortion of a person is morally permissible.

7.4 Critical Analysis of the Violinist Analogy

7.4.1 *The Misunderstood Samaritan*

The strength of Thomson's violinist analogy rests on the intuition that you may "unplug" yourself from the violinist, but this intuition may be considerably weakened by her appeal to the story of the Good Samaritan. If we follow Thomson in using the parable of the Good Samaritan to enlighten the case at hand, we can understand the meaning of the story better by considering its context. The story of the Good Samaritan is occasioned by a question posed to Jesus by a lawyer about how we should act. Jesus affirms, "'Love the Lord your God with all your heart and with all your soul and with all your strength and with all your mind;' and, 'Love your neighbor as yourself.'" These imperatives are commands about what is required to do (at least it would seem in the view of Jesus), rather than what would be supererogatory, above and beyond the call of duty, to do (such as selling all one's possessions and giving the money to the poor). After Jesus confirms the duty to love God and neighbor, the lawyer then asks, "Who is my neighbor?" a question which prompts the story of the Good Samaritan. After telling the story, and indicting that the Good Samaritan was neighbor to the person in need, Jesus says, "Go and do likewise." The context of the story, both before and after the parable itself, indicates that loving neighbor is not merely a matter of going above and beyond the call of duty, but rather is a moral requirement.

Thomson is aware of this interpretation of the parable, "Perhaps he [Jesus] meant that we are morally required to act as the Good Samaritan did" (Thomson 1971, p. 63). In response to this consideration, Thomson emphasizes that the law normally does not compel us to act as Good Samaritans (though laws drafting citizens into the military defense of a country may serve as a counter example). However, the point of the parable seems to be not a *legal* one, but rather a *moral* one. We should—in an ethical sense of should—help those in need even though the law may not compel us to do so. Since this book addresses the ethical and not the legal question of abortion, even if Thomson is correct about what the law holds or what the law ought to be, it may still be ethically required to help those in need. The fact that we do not know the stranger, and that we did not bring about his neediness, is irrelevant. Anyone in need whom I can help is my neighbor. This interpretation accords well with the ethic generally proposed by Jesus. We are commanded to love our neighbor as ourselves, and care especially for those who are the most weak and disadvantaged, for example, the poor, the leper, the outcast, the unwanted. I am not making an argument from religious authority in order to point to the immorality of abortion. Of course, *if* someone is going to follow the teachings of Jesus, then the views of Jesus are authoritative in terms guiding conduct. My point, as I take it was Thomson's, is to appeal to the wisdom contained in the parable, just as one might appeal to the parables of Aesop, Confucius, or any other figure. If this interpretation of the parable is correct, then using the parable of the Good Samaritan to justify not helping someone in need is rather like using the story of the race between the tortoise and the hare to justify a lack of perseverance or the tale of the three little pigs who built houses of straw, sticks, and bricks to justify playing rather than doing your work well.

7.4.2 The Bodily Integrity Objection

But one need not assume the wisdom of this reading of the Good Samaritan parable in order to find fault with Thomson's analogy. Unplugging suggests that in causing a separation between you and the violinist, you are not doing anything to the bodily integrity of the violinist himself.

You are perhaps snipping the cord that connects the two of you, but not actually doing anything to the violinist's own body.

Consider the violinist analogy again, with the "unplugging" replaced by a means of freeing yourself from the violinist that impinges on his bodily integrity and induces his death. Imagine for instance that you are to separate yourself from the violinist by poisoning him or by taking an ax to his body or by tearing him limb from limb or by putting him through an incredibly powerful suction machine (akin to a jet engine, say) that would leave him in recognizable pieces on the other side. If we were to separate ourselves from the violinist by any of *these* means, then things begin to look quite a bit different. We are not simply separating ourselves or cutting a cord that links us to the violinist. Rather, we are doing something to the body of the violinist who, if he is a person, has as much right to bodily integrity as do we.

In addition, if such violent means were used, the death of the violinist would not come about because of his own underlying pathology. In these cases, the violinist dies because *we*, or our agents, not only cause but also apparently intend his death through the various means. So the strength of Thomson's analogy will inevitably depend in part on what methods are actually used for abortion. Is abortion more like unplugging or more like chopping up?

To answer this question requires us to examine the various ways abortions are performed. What are the methods of abortion commonly used? Stephanie D. Schmutz has given a description of the most commonly used methods of abortion, namely: Suction curettage, dilation and evacuation, dilation and extraction or partial-birth abortion, and induction:

> *Suction curettage.* Vacuum aspiration abortion or suction curettage is the most common form of surgical abortion in the first trimester of pregnancy and normally involves either local or general anesthesia. After dilating the cervix, the physician uses a powerful suction machine to remove part by part the contents of the uterus, until the human fetus and placenta are entirely outside the womb.

> *Dilation and evacuation.* D & E is the most common method for second trimester abortions and involves an overnight dilation of the cervix, using seaweed to slowly open the entrance to the uterus. Following the dilation of the cervix, the doctor evacuates the contents of the uterus using suction and forceps to dismember the developing human being in order to remove the human fetus more easily from the uterus.

> *Dilation and extraction* or *partial-birth abortion* is similar to the D & E, with the exception that the D & X involves a partial breach delivery of the human fetus prior to the abortion and may be used in

the second or third trimester of pregnancy. After the woman's cervix has been dilated, the physician uses forceps to locate the human fetus's lower extremities (such as a foot or leg). The physician then uses his hands partially to deliver the fetus, being careful however not to deliver the head. The doctor then reduces the size of the head so it can also pass through the cervix by piercing the skull of the human fetus's head with scissors and inserting a tube into the head to suction out the brain and other cranial contents. (Schmutz 2002, p. 552)

Induction. Used in the second and third trimester, induction involves injecting the amniotic cavity in the uterus with a hypertonic solution of urea, prostaglandin, or saline. These solutions kill the human fetus and induce contractions, which result in delivery.

The critic of the violinist argument would point out that each of these forms of abortion fails rather grossly to resemble the delicate separation suggested by "unplugging." All these forms of abortion directly attack the body of the human fetus and directly induce fetal death. Admittedly, there is some plausibility to the idea that we can separate ourselves from the violinist, allowing him to die. However, it would be considerably less plausible to argue that we could be morally justified in causing the separation by means of tearing his body limb from limb by means of a powerful vacuum (as in suction abortion), taking an ax to his or her body or head (in a manner reminiscent of D&C and D&X abortions), or poisoning him or her (as in induction abortions). In some cases, the violinist may be conscious (later abortion) and in other cases not conscious (early abortion), but the additional factor of causing pain only compounds the greater wrongdoing of intentionally undermining the bodily integrity of a person. As McMahan frankly admits, "The standard methods for performing abortions clearly involve killing the fetus: the fetus dies by being mangled or poisoned in the process of being removed from the uterus" (2002, p. 378).

A defender of the violinist argument could respond that not all forms of abortion actually kill and undermine the bodily integrity of the human fetus. Although they are rarely used, there are two forms of abortion that do closely resemble unplugging, namely hysterotomy and hysterectomy. Hysterotomy or Cesarean section takes place when the human fetus is surgically delivered through an incision in the uterine wall and abdomen. If the human fetus were not yet viable, then this removal would lead to fetal death, which would be caused by what might be construed as the underlying pathology of the human fetus, underdeveloped lungs. This form of abortion is rarely used because of an increased danger to maternal health. The same holds true for hysterectomy, which removes the entire uterus of the mother, rendering her infertile and, if the human fetus is not viable, leading to the death of the young human being. If forms of abortion were used which did not directly attack the body of the prenatal human being, and death resulted from, say, underdeveloped lung capacity, then one could not criticize the violinist analogy for failing to capture two relevant factors in the way abortions are usually performed: (1) there is a direct intervention against the body of the fetal human, and (2) the death of the human being in utero is directly caused by this intervention. Even in such cases, and even if the death is not sought intentionally, it is still morally required that one has a proportionately serious reason for allowing the death of one's own offspring (or at least this will be argued in the next chapter in section 8.1.5), and aside from, for example, the case of trying to save the life of the mother, this proportionately serious reason for allowing the death of the offspring is not present.

7.4.3 The Consistency Objection

However, even if such methods of abortion were in fact the ones used, another problem with the violinist analogy would remain. Since the violinist and you are equally persons, let's consider the scenario from the violinist's perspective. It is true you didn't choose to be hooked up to him, but it is equally true that he didn't choose to be hooked up to you. Let's imagine that the violinist does not like being hooked up to you. Suppose further that he has spotted another person, who also could support him, a person he finds extremely attractive and charming. In ways too numerous to list, he finds her exciting to be near and, frankly, he has grown weary of being plugged into you. Moreover, being hooked up to *you* is, in his estimation, a serious burden. Unfortunately, technology being what it presently is, the violinist cannot simply snip the cord that links you to himself. Indeed, in order to separate himself from you, he will end up causing *your* death, though he would survive by being immediately hooked up to the person he likes better. (Like being hooked up to the violinists in the first place, we can only speculate how this happens. We could also change the case by saying that it is not another person he gets hooked up to but a newly invented machine.) The violinist would prefer that you not die, and sadly your death would be an unfortunate side effect of unplugging, but it would not be right to force *him* to be a Good Samaritan just to keep you alive for nine months. Would it be morally permissible for him to detach himself from you, if the only way to do so would involve your death? After all, if *you* may unplug yourself from the violinist, causing his death, then *he* should also be able to unplug himself from you, causing your death. Things tend to look a little different from this perspective, and our intuitions change. The violinist, it would seem, is not justified in unplugging himself from you causing your death.

But if the violinist may not unplug himself from you causing your death, then it is only fair that you not unplug yourself from him causing his death. If so, then unplugging, even true unplugging that doesn't intentionally undermine the bodily integrity of the other person directly causing his or her death, is not justified after all.

It might be objected, however, that the golden rule is not best applied by asking how I would like it if X did to me what I am considering doing to X under the present circumstances, but whether I would object to X doing that to me if I was in X's circumstances. I can make my students unhappy with a justified bad grade, but I don't recognize the justice of that by asking whether they can make *me* unhappy with a justified bad grade. So, are there differences in circumstance that make the violinists unplugging from me wrong, but make it permissible for me to unplug myself from him?

There are, of course, a number of differences between the modified case of the violinist and the case of pregnancy, but it is not clear these are morally relevant. Even though the human fetus lacks the power to detach, the question is about the *moral right* to detach from the mother at the cost of the mother's life. Although a human fetus is not powerful enough to detach itself from the mother, an agent acting on behalf of the human fetus is certainly powerful enough. Indeed, in a typical case of abortion, a woman does not induce the abortion herself but someone acting on her behalf does.

Another difference a defender of the violinist argument could make is that you are benefiting the violinist who has a kidney dysfunction and the violinist is not benefiting you, so perhaps this difference would justify you unplugging from him and make his unplugging from you unjustified. Since the mother benefits the human fetus, and the human fetus does not benefit the mother, the mother has a right to disconnect herself from the human fetus but the human fetus does not have the right to disconnect from the mother.

Although a "one way" benefit is present in some pregnancies, this is not true of all pregnancies. It can happen for instance that the mother is not providing any *necessary* benefit to the fetal human being as at the very end of pregnancy at which point the human being in utero could survive quite well ex utero. (It should be noted that some defenders of abortion do indeed hold that abortion is impermissible after the point of viability, but as was argued earlier there is no good reason to think that viability makes any difference in the moral status of the fetus (section 4.1.2). Defenders of the violinist argument may accept this same conclusion for different reasons).

In other cases, the mother not only does not provide a necessary benefit to the child but also undermines the well-being of the human fetus, as is the case of heavy alcohol or drug abuse late in pregnancy when the human fetus would be better off being born. Furthermore, if abortion is going to be performed, then the woman no longer intends to benefit her progeny. So, it is not always the case that the pregnant woman provides a necessary benefit or is going to continue to benefit.

Sometimes there is a two-way benefit in pregnancy, the mother benefiting the human fetus and the human fetus benefiting the mother. There is evidence that continuing with a pregnancy benefits women with breast cancer more than having an abortion would (Clark & Chua 1989). There is also evidence that likelihood of suicide is greater when a pregnancy is aborted rather than carried to term (Jansson 1965; Gissler, Hemminki, & Lonnqvist 1996). Women suffering from MS report an alleviation of MS symptoms during pregnancy. Many women report other physical and psychological benefits during pregnancy. So, even if the benefit in the violinist example goes only from you to the violinist, benefits (and harms) in actual pregnancies are not always simply one way from mother to progeny. To make the violinist argument more like pregnancy we could stipulate that sometimes the one hooked up to the violinist provides no necessary benefit to the violinist, sometimes he or she actually harms or is about to harm the violinist, and sometimes the violinist provides physical and/or psychological benefit to the person with whom he is hooked up. So we arrive at the same conclusion. Since the violinist may not unplug himself from you at the cost of your life, you may not unplug yourself from him at the cost of his life. Analogously, since the human fetus (acting through another agent) may not unplug from the mother at the cost of the woman's life, the woman (normally acting through another agent) may not unplug from the human fetus at the cost of fetal life.

Does the consistency objection simply beg the question at issue? Thomson's analogy is meant to underscore the point that it is permissible to unplug yourself from the violinist because the violinist is making use of something that the violinist does not have a right to make use of. But in the case described, your being alive is not the result of your making use of what you had no right to use.

But surely, if there were cases—similar to the MS case where the human fetus benefits the mother—in which the fetus actually kept the woman alive, this would not give the human fetus grounds for killing the mother by some agent. Imagine that becoming pregnant would cure a woman in the last stages of dying from AIDS. We would then have a case of the fetus keeping the woman alive. Surely, however, whether a woman has AIDS and whether AIDS is cured by pregnancy is irrelevant to whether abortion is wrong. In some cases of proposed capital punishment, the existence of the human fetus preserves the life of the mother because the woman's life is temporarily or permanently spared from the death penalty solely on the grounds that she is pregnant and a mother. In such cases, an agent acting privately on behalf of the human fetus would not be justified in disconnecting the human being in utero from the mother at the cost of her life. Indeed, simply asserting that the fetus is making use of that to which he or she has no right itself seems to beg the question. After all, critics of the violinist argument believe that the woman has a duty towards the fetus, so in accepting benefit from the mother the child is receiving that which he or she has a right to receive.

7.4.4 The Intention/Foresight Objection

Other problems have been raised for violinist argument. The analogy relies on our intuition that death that is merely foreseen and not intended, allowed but not chosen, may sometimes be justified. Unplugging in the violinist analogy suggests that the death of the violinist results from *his* illness rather than as an effect *you* intended. You were, by being hooked up to him, forestalling his death, which you foresaw would take place if you did not remain plugged into him. Recall that the violinist has an underlying pathology and would die without your help. So when you "unplug" yourself from the violinist it is rather akin to a medical team not taking extraordinary measures to save someone's life. The team certainly may use such measures, they may go above and beyond the call of duty to try to save human life, but there is no obligation to do so. Likewise, you certainly could have saved the violinist but, since you didn't go the extra mile, he will die from his own illness. Put another way, the analogy suggests that the death of the violinist is a foreseen but not intended result of your action, and often we can justify causing death to others in such cases. But it is hard to imagine that the forms of abortion most frequently used (suction curettage, dilation and evacuation, dilation and extraction or partial-birth abortion, and induction) do not constitute intentional killing.

Some attempt to shore up the violinist argument by claiming that there is no important moral difference between intending some effect and merely foreseeably causing it. On this view, there is no moral difference between intending some effect and not intending but merely causing and foreseeing that some effect may come about as a result of a chosen action. So, if it is permissible merely to foresee that the death of the violinist will come about as a result of your action, it is also morally permissible to intentionally kill to achieve the same effect. (It is important to emphasize that the distinction between intention and foresight is not the same as the distinction between doing and allowing. One can intentionally allow some evil effect.)

The view that the distinction between intending and foreseeably causing is unimportant morally, however, should be rejected. A general may fully foresee that some of his soldiers will be killed in battle, but he does not intend their deaths. In a just war, he accepts the foreseen deaths of his troops for the proportionately serious reason of securing a just peace, including the saving of the lives of innocent civilians. On the other hand, a tyrant might kill some of his own troops intentionally in order to scare his other troops into absolute obedience or in order to make it appear that the enemy is ruthless and thereby motivate his troops to fight more fiercely. Or, the tyrant may simply view his soldiers as expendable means. Although an equal number of troops might die in both cases, the general and the tyrant differ radically. Killing that is accepted as an unfortunate but unavoidable side effect of action needed to achieve an important good is one thing; killing the innocent as a means or as an end in itself (that is, intentionally bringing about the death of innocent human beings) is quite another.

The distinction between intention and foresight illuminates many other examples, as well: Consider the difference between the kindly dentist who merely foresees, and regrets, that a tooth removal will cause pain and the sadistic dentist who is intending that a tooth removal cause pain. So other things being equal, if X effect is bad, it is worse to intend X than merely to foreseeably cause X. Put another way, if X is an evil effect, it is harder to justify intending X than merely foreseeably causing X. So at least in some cases, it may be morally permissible to foreseeably cause X, but it may not be morally permissible to intend X. For example, sociologists note a relationship between education and suicide. The more education a person has, the more likely it is that he or she will commit suicide. So, if a society promotes education, a predictable side effect will be the increased incidence of suicide. Although promotion of education involves an increase in human death as an unforeseen side effect, it may still be morally justified to accept such a bad side effect rather than deny people an opportunity at higher education because the effect is unintended. (However, this differs entirely from an attempt to justify killing human beings in order not to deny others an opportunity at higher education. Say you know your rich neighbors have planned in their wills to donate fortunes to the local university after their death to establish scholarships for needy students. It would obviously be impermissible to kill them so as to provide others with scholarship money.) In the vast majority of cases where abortion is desired, the actual condition of pregnancy is not the chief perceived problem but rather the responsibility for the child that ensues from birth. Hence, most abortions are undertaken precisely in order to end the developing human life. Characteristically, those seeking an abortion want the human fetus not to exist; they do not want merely a cessation of the pregnancy. In the words of Leslie Cannold, "What women intend in choosing abortion is not only to terminate their pregnancy, but to end *the life of their fetus*" (Cannold 2000, p. 60, emphasis in the original). In fact, a woman might want *both* to end the pregnancy *and* to end the life of the human fetus, having two intentions in the act, either one of which alone might be sufficient.

If, however, the intention to end the life is present, then even if other sufficient intentions are also present, the act, as defined by intention, would be direct abortion. It is possible for an act, considered from the exterior point of view, to have two proper moral characterizations based on two intentions. Taking some compromising photos out of someone's desk drawer, which he had hidden there, could constitute both stealing from that person and violating privacy. If the action were not stealing but merely violating privacy, the action would still be wrong. If one of the intentions is licit, but the other is not, the action would still be wrong, since all the defining aspects of an action must be right for the action to be right. This thesis that all the aspects of an action must be right for the action to be right as a whole may be somewhat controversial itself. I have elsewhere offered some considerations in defense of it (Kaczor 2002). Briefly, moral goodness is lacking if any aspect of what ought to be there is missing. If someone is missing benevolent motivations, then the action in question (taken as a whole) is lacking something it ought to have, and so is not morally good. In any case, critics of the violinist argument have argued that one reason unplugging from the violinist is acceptable, but abortions are not, is that in the case of the violinist the death is foreseen, but in the case of abortion fetal death is intended.

Boonin has provided an objection to this line of argument by applying an account of the importance and parsing of the intention/foresight distinction suggested by Warren Quinn (1989). To simplify the examples Boonin gives (2003, p. 223), imagine two bombers A and B who have a legitimate target, a munitions factory, in a just war. Suppose bomber A has a newly developed bomb that for technical reasons cannot be successfully detonated in the presence of living human beings. So, finding some civilians who happen to be sleeping on the roof of the factory, he first kills them and then drops his new bomb on the factory. This is akin to intentional killing or direct abortion. Bomber B doesn't intentionally kill the civilians first before bombing the munitions plant, though regrettably, they die during the bombing, but as a result he places himself in much greater danger, since the civilians can, before they die, notify others who can then shoot at Bomber B. Bomber B's actions are akin to indirect abortion—like hysterectomy of a gravid cancerous uterus. Everyone agrees that the action of Bomber B is permissible. But if this is granted then Bomber A's actions should also be permissible, for two reasons (Boonin 2003, p. 223). First, Bomber A would not kill the civilians if there were some possible situation in which he could obtain the goal without killing, Bomber A is not violating the purpose of the intention/foresight distinction, which precludes using persons as if they exist for your own purposes. Second,

> [I]f Bomber [A] chooses to gas the sleeping civilians and then drop Bomb A, he does not choose intentionally causing death over not causing death. Rather, he chooses intentionally causing death over foreseeably causing death, in a context where the choice between the two makes no difference to the ones who will die but does make a difference to him in terms of the degree of risk of harm he will face. This is a fundamentally different kind of choice.
>
> (Boonin 2003, p. 224)

Bomber A and Bomber B both cause the death of civilians, and since causing the death of the civilians is not in itself impermissible, and since the way in which they die makes no difference to the civilians, Bomber A's decision is permissible. It is an acceptable choice since it preserves the only good which can be preserved in this situation, namely not placing the bomber in greater danger than he needs to be in order to obtain his legitimate goal. So if Bomber B's action is acceptable, then Bomber A's action is too.

One possible objection to this argument would be to deny Quinn's account of intention, on which the argument depends (Marquis 1991; Fischer, Ravizza, & Copp 1993). But Boonin's argument requires not only that Quinn's account is correct, but also that other (compatible) accounts of the intention/foresight distinction must be mistaken, such as those provided by, for example, Cavanaugh (1996), Finnis, Grisez, and Boyle (2001), or Aulisio (1996). Boonin does not show that such alternative accounts are mistaken, but rather he argues that Thomson's analogy is compatible with some accounts of the intention/foresight distinction such as Quinn's.

But even if Quinn's account of the moral importance of the distinction were accepted, and even if it were the only justification for the distinction, the counter-factual way of accounting for the purpose of the intention/foresight distinction is problematic. Even if it is true that Bomber A would destroy the munitions plant without having to kill the civilians, if he could, it hardly follows that he does not use their deaths for his own purposes. Let's say a woman has legitimate reason to want a man not to reveal an important secret of hers, a secret that if known would ruin her social standing and political career. He says that he is going to reveal it anyway, and she has every reason to believe that he will. She decides to kill him as the only way to make sure that her important secret remains safe. If there were any other way to make sure he would not reveal this secret, she would use it. Unfortunately, such methods don't exist and the only way to ensure his silence on this matter is to kill him. Although the woman really would not kill him if any other options were available, she nevertheless uses his death as a means to her end and does not view the man as if he exists for his own purposes. So even if an agent would not choose direct abortion if other options were available, the agent nevertheless uses the death of the fetus as a means to the agent's end and treats the human fetus as if he or she exists for the agent's own purposes.

Let us alter this case so that it even more closely mirrors the case of Bomber A and Bomber B. Imagine this woman is flying a helicopter with this man as her only passenger deep in the South Pacific. Their helicopter crashes, and they are stuck on a deserted island. This island has searing heat during the day and wild tropical storms with freezing rain at night. They use the helicopter as the only available shelter from the intense, inhospitable weather which would kill them in less than a single day if they were exposed. Due to the crash, the helicopter only has enough fuel to fly one person at very slow speed to the nearest island more than a full day away, and only the woman knows how to fly helicopters. She now faces a choice. She could kill him before she leaves to preserve her secret or, taking away the helicopter, she could just leave him without any means of communication on a desert island, fully foreseeing that he will die of exposure before anyone can rescue him. If she just leaves him to die by depriving him of shelter, he could possibly put a message in a bottle, which someone might find, revealing her secret. So, before she flies away, she shoots him to death rather than risking him revealing the secret. She does something seriously wrong, even though her escaping the island would have resulted in his death as a foreseen side effect anyway. The woman chooses intentionally killing over foreseeably causing death, in a context where the choice between the two makes no difference to the one who will die but does make a difference to her in terms of the degree of risk of harm she will face. Despite the circumstances, she has made a fundamentally immoral kind of choice in shooting the man.

Likewise, Bomber A chooses to kill innocent persons intentionally as a an extra means to secure his safety. Bomber B avoids intentionally killing innocent persons and, therefore, puts himself at greater risk. If intentional killing of an innocent person is wrong, then the fact that someone who does not do wrong must take greater risks in achieving his objective than does someone who is willing to do wrong, is merely a reminder that doing what's right is not always easy. One lesson from Plato in the *Crito* is that abstaining from wrongdoing can be costly. The intention/foresight distinction is meant to determine what aspects of the effects of an action constitute one's choice, and so the fact that abstaining from choosing evil involves a greater risk to an agent would not thereby make the choice to do evil in such circumstances into a different kind of choice.

Some abortions, however, may not fall into the category of killing as a means or as an end. Imagine a model who wants to terminate her pregnancy, not because she fears the responsibility a newborn would entail (whether through raising the child or through placing the child in another family through adoption) but because it is the condition of pregnancy itself she wishes to avoid. It is not that she wishes to destroy the human fetus but rather that she seeks to avoid being pregnant which, at least in later stages, would endanger her svelte figure. Although some fashion magazines do cater to pregnant women, one seldom sees a woman near the end of pregnancy on the catwalk. Imagine further that the method of abortion is hysterotomy or hysterectomy, so that the body of the human fetus will be removed or "unplugged" from the mother rather than directly destroyed.

In response to this variation of the violinist argument, a critic may argue that surely such an agent does in fact intend the death of the fetus.

After all, the means chosen to preserve her figure from enlarging is to stop the growing of the human fetus by means of killing him or her, and whatever is chosen as a means is intended.

Even if somehow the death of the human fetus was not intended, the model aborting to preserve her figure accepts an evil consequence that is grossly disproportionate to the good preserved. It is wrong to accept, even as an unintended side effect, such a significant harm to another for the sake of a less significant good. For example, Patrick Lee cites the example of a father who works and lives near a plant producing massive amounts of toxic chemicals. Even though his work situation gravely harms his daughter, he refuses to change jobs because to do so would disadvantage him professionally. In fact, he is willing to accept the death of his child rather than incur such professional disadvantage. In Lee's words,

> If he does not use the chemicals he simply must get a new career. He tells his wife he is sorry but their child will just have to die, because he will not change his career. Here we would say that change in occupation is not comparable to a child's death. Even though in both actions there is a harm to a real and basic human good, still, the fact that shifting careers is not as total and irreparable a loss as death makes the action unjust or unfair.
>
> (1996, p. 117)

Surely, such a father acts wrongly, and hence so would a mother who chooses an "indirect abortion," of the sort described in the next chapter, without a proportionately serious reason.

But let us return to the analogies. Thomson offers more than just the violinist argument in justifying abortion. Does Thomson's burglar analogy demonstrate the moral permissibility of abortion, and thus succeed where the violinist analogy fails? Critics have pointed out several disanalogies between the burglar case and abortion.

7.5 Critical Analysis of the Burglar Analogy

The critic of the burglar analogy could critique the analogy by pointing out that the woman's action of leaving the door unlocked does not cause the burglar to be in the house—opening the door only removes an obstacle. On the other hand, the man and the woman cause the baby to be where it is, even if they tried to prevent it (just as a drunk driver causes deaths though she may have tried to prevent it, say by drinking coffee to help stay alert). In Lee's words,

> Parents have a special duty or responsibility to their children even if they have taken careful precautions to avoid having children, by contraception or natural family planning. For most people realize

that contraceptives and other methods of avoiding conception have a certain rate of failure. Similarly, drunk drivers are responsible for the damage they cause even if they make great efforts to avoid it. If the baseball I bat breaks my neighbor's window, I still have a responsibility to compensate my neighbor (fix the window) even though I tried very hard to bat the baseball in the other direction. Thus, contrary to Thomson's argument, we *are* responsible for the natural and foreseen results of our actions even if we try to avoid them.

(1996, p. 118, emphasis in the original)

Boonin critiques this argument by drawing a distinction between being responsible for someone's existence and being responsible for someone's neediness given that the person exists. Let's say I enjoy playing with fire and foresee that lighting a fire here and now may lead to a blaze that could destroy your house. I light the fire and indeed it does destroy your house. Since I am responsible for your neediness, I owe you restitution. However, "where you are responsible for the needy person's existence but not for his neediness, given that he exists—the individual in need has not acquired the right to your assistance. And if this is so, then the responsibility objection fails" (Boonin 2003, p. 174). Since there was no situation in which the woman could have conceived without having the conceived being also be needy, the woman is responsible for the existence of the human fetus but not for its neediness and therefore she is not obliged to help.

Boonin asks us to imagine that a doctor gave a patient an "imperfect drug" needed to save his life, but as a possible side effect, the drug would some years later render the patient in the same situation as the violinist. Unfortunately, the patient does indeed end up in a situation similar to the violinist. In such a case, would the doctor, since he is responsible for the patient's existence, also have a duty to be hooked up to the patient for nine months while the patient recovered? No, the doctor would not have any such duty. The doctor is responsible for the existence of the patient but, since there was no way to save the patient without risking the side effect, he is not responsible for the neediness of the patient and so has no duty to be hooked up to him.

A critic of Boonin's imperfect drug argument could respond that the analogy between the mother and the doctor doesn't really work in the first place. Unlike the mother, the doctor *isn't* really responsible for the other person's *existence* per se, but only for the other person's *being healed* (which obviously means that the person must have *already* existed in order to be healed). Boonin does note in his book (2003, pp. 169, 170) that "responsible for existence" should be understood as responsible for the fact that a person *now* exists, that is, continues to exist but this is no different in meaning than saying that the doctor is responsible for the patient's remaining healthy (which, again, is different than being responsible for the existence of the being in itself).

Another difficulty with this argument is that, in the case of pregnancy, it would seem to prove too much. Since a mother is responsible only for the existence and not the neediness of the human fetus, the woman has no duty to provide assistance to her progeny in utero even if failing to provide assistance leads to the death of the progeny. But then it would also follow that taking crack cocaine throughout pregnancy is not morally problematic. After all, the pregnant woman taking crack cocaine may be responsible for the *existence* of the human fetus within her, but she is not responsible for the *neediness* of the human fetus in terms of the fetus's susceptibility to being damaged by cocaine abuse. The same holds true for abusing alcohol or other drugs. If there is no duty to aid when even life and death are on the line, then there is no duty to aid when the psychological or physical well-being of a human fetus hangs in the balance. Put differently, if you do not have a responsibility to prevent someone from dying, *a fortiori* you do not have a responsibility to prevent lesser harms to that person. If you may harm someone even to the point of death, it is also permissible to inflict lesser harms on the person. If the violinist analogy permits abortion, even more so would this reasoning make the use of crack during pregnancy morally permissible, which does not kill but merely injures the prenatal person.

But let's return to other critiques of the burglar analogy. A second disanalogy between the burglar and a human fetus is that a burglar enters a person's house under his own power. Having done something wrong, he does not merit our sympathy. If a burglar breaks into your house, he is knowingly and willingly breaking the law and violating your privacy. The burglar, being guilty, forfeits some of the rights enjoyed by an innocent person. But suppose that the "burglar" was involuntarily in the house. Say a 2-year-old child or an elderly grandma with dementia wanders accidentally into the house. Not only does she not knowingly violate anyone's property rights but also she doesn't even realize where she is. Would it be acceptable to kill such a person, an unwitting trespasser, if this were the only way to make the person leave the house? Mary Anne Warren answers this question negatively.

> Mere ownership does not give me the right to kill innocent people whom I find on my property, and indeed I am apt to be held responsible if such people injure themselves while on my property. It is equally unclear that I have any moral right to expel an innocent person from my property when I know that doing so will result in his death.
>
> (1996, p. 80)

The human fetus, on the other hand, is according to Thomson's concession for the sake of argument an innocent person at least formally speaking since the human fetus is not trying to cause any harm. Indeed, the human fetus could not be voluntarily doing wrong, since a human being at this stage of development does not have a developed capacity for responsibility and will not have such capacity in any sense at all until after the age of two at the very earliest. Indeed, the "age of reason," or the age at which children are sometimes said to begin to be responsible for their actions, is often held to begin around eight years of age. So even if one has a right to expel a guilty burglar from one's house, this would not mean that one also has the right to expel an innocent human being from the womb. We are morally justified in treating the guilty in ways we are not morally justified in treating the innocent. Small immature human beings in particular merit our kindness and consideration, rather than our wrath should they unknowingly be where we would prefer that they not be.

A third disanalogy that could be raised against the burglar analogy is that just leaving windows or doors open does not in itself lead to burglars (or people seeds) entering the house in the way that having sexual intercourse leads to pregnancy. Suppose that leaving doors unlocked often led to young children or elderly neighbors wandering innocently into your house. Suppose we spoke of leaving doors ajar as the "neighbor-inviting act," just as we speak of sexual intercourse as the generative act or reproductive act. Suppose further that you *caused* the child or elderly neighbor to be in your house, say by grabbing a child or an octogenarian who looked very much like your own niece or grandma off the street and dragging the person into your house. Even if you couldn't find another way of getting her out of your house as quickly as you'd like, you would hardly be justified in killing her, because she is in your house *only* because of your *own* actions. Contrary to what McDonagh argues in *Breaking the Abortion Deadlock* the critic of the burglar analogy could argue that the human fetus cannot "be held accountable" for what it does, since the human fetus cannot exercise responsibility any more than can a newborn baby. Those who have responsibility to ensure the well-being of the human fetus are those who caused the fetus to be where it is, namely the parents. Of course, Thomson denies that the biological ties lead to responsibilities, which brings us to the question of special responsibilities.

7.6 Special Duties to Care for Children?

As mentioned earlier, Thomson recognizes that parents have duties to their own children that strangers do not have to anonymous violinists, burglars, or floating people-plants. To be a minimally decent parent, one must do many things that if done to strangers would constitute being a Good Samaritan, indeed a Splendid Samaritan. However, Thomson denies that special duties arise from biological parent–child relationship. A pregnant woman does not have duties to her progeny in utero, says

Thomson, because she has not implicitly or explicitly assumed special responsibility for the child which do not come into existence through a mere biological relationship (Thomson 1971, p. 65).

Is it really reasonable to assume, as Thomson's argument does, that special responsibilities to a person exist *only* if explicitly or implicitly assumed? Consider the relationship of adult children to parents. It would seem fairly clear that adult children *do* have special responsibilities for their parents simply in virtue of their biological relationship. Many well-known stories hinge on the importance of such biological relationships, even if not initially known. Moses discovers he is a Hebrew rather than a prince of Egypt. Oedipus, not realizing their identities, kills his father and marries his mother. Luke Skywalker learns that his father is Darth Vader. Indeed, such stories make little sense without presupposing that biological relationships are morally, *humanly* important, and not just because we *decide* they are important.

If someone were to fail to care properly for his or her elderly mother, and when confronted were to say: "Of course, I have neglected my mother. But I never explicitly or implicitly took responsibility for her, so I owe her nothing more than I owe a stranger." This excuse would compound the wrongdoing rather than excuse it. Obviously, the responsibilities of adult children to parents vary according to the situation. It could in fact be a responsible act, in some circumstances, to ignore a parent, even for long stretches of time. However, it would not be true, even in this case, that our responsibility for them is just the same as our responsibility to a stranger unless we voluntarily assume it. Similar remarks could be made about the special responsibilities *siblings* have towards one another. We don't choose our brother or sister, but nevertheless we have special responsibilities for our siblings that we do not have to strangers, and these duties plainly do not arise simply from our implicit or explicit assumption of such duties. Partly for this reason, patricide, matricide, and fratricide are viewed as especially vicious because love is due particularly to parents and siblings precisely on account of this family relationship, one that is not created by our choosing (though in the case of adoption and voluntary procreation it is created by another person's choosing).

Nor is the importance of biological relationships limited to parents and siblings: it also extends to children. If mothers do not have a special responsibility for their children by virtue of their biological relationship, then the same lack of duty should hold true for fathers. Such a view would have profound moral and legal consequences. If Thomson's view is right, then fathers would owe no child support to the women they impregnate (unless they choose to take responsibility for their children) because a man's biological relationship to his child would in no way entail that he has a special responsibility for it. This would be particularly true if the man used contraception. But of course legal and moral duties of paternity do not depend on such circumstances. No man has ever justly evaded child support payments by pleading "the condom broke."

What if the biological father will participate in creating the child only on condition that he not have to pay child support or will not have to give any aid whatsoever to the child? One can think of a sperm donor or perhaps someone who says, "I just want to let you know, if you get pregnant, you are on your own. I will not help you or any child of ours in any way." Would such a biological father still have duties to his child?

Such men, it seems to me, are cads of the highest order, but even cads have duties. One's duties to one's own offspring cannot be bartered away by fiat of the father, or the mother, or both father and mother together. In conceiving a child, both biological parents likewise conceive duties towards their child, and the despicable conduct of one parent or both does not void these responsibilities. What is of paramount importance is the well-being of the vulnerable child, not of the parents.

Biological fathers have a special responsibility for their children, simply in virtue of having begotten their offspring. Consider for a moment what is typically involved in a man's taking responsibility for a child he has begotten merely from a financial perspective. The burdens of child support are considerable and vary with the income of the father. In 2002, the average support paid to children under 21 was $350 per month (Grall 2005, p. 1). Over the course of the years and until the child turns eighteen (though sometimes payments continue until twenty-one or later), he can expect to pay $75,600. Translated into work hours, for many people this would be income for more than two full years of employment. A failure to fulfill this obligation can result in prison time.

Just as the burdens of paying child support vary from father to father, so too the burdens of pregnancy differ in various cases. However, we do have some idea how burdensome pregnancy is, at least as measured financially, from the experience of surrogate mothers. "Gestational carriers," as they sometimes prefer to be called, are paid on average between $20,000 to $25,000 dollars (Ali and Kelley 2008). In other words, the average father paying child support undertakes a burden—measured financially—that is greater over time than the average burden undertaken in pregnancy.

Of course, to be a *minimally* decent father, he must do much more than send a monthly check. He must contribute to her well-being, either by securing loving parents for her via adoption or by providing for her himself. If he does not choose to discharge his parental duties in the first way, he must do a great deal to be a minimally decent father. For example, he should also attend her athletic events, inspect report cards, listen to piano practice, teach her to ride a bike, take her swimming, etc. *Above all*, he should refrain from harming her, even if harming her is to his apparent advantage.

Since this is true for men, simply in virtue of having begotten a child, it is fair that women (whether biological mothers or gestational mothers), too, should have similar duties. If they do not discharge their duty by securing that the child's needs are met by others (adoption), then they must do it themselves. Indeed the burdens of being a minimally decent father or mother would seem much greater than the typical burdens of pregnancy. The vast majority of women, for most of the duration of a pregnancy, need not be consciously *doing anything* in order to *provide everything* that the human fetus needs to thrive. A pregnant woman could be sound asleep, exercising, writing a paper, chatting with a friend, and at the same time be providing all that is needed for the well-being of her progeny in utero. However, following birth, fathers and mothers will be called upon, if they are to be minimally decent, let alone good, fathers and mothers, to *do* a great many things. (One possible option at this point is adoption by which the parents fully discharge and terminate their parental duties by securing adoptive parents to care for the child.) An unconscious person could function perfectly well as a gestational mother, but an unconscious person could not begin to function as a minimally decent social parent, the one who socializes the children and cares for the child's everyday needs. Normally of course being a gestational mother does involve substantial burdens, but being a minimally decent social parent normally involves substantially greater burdens. Since the moral obligations of being a minimally decent father are normally greater than the burdens of being a minimally decent gestational mother, and since morality requires that fathers aid their children, critics of Thomson's analogies have argued that it makes sense that gestational mothers also provide aid.

7.7 The Comparative Burdens Objection

The inherently unequal burdens of gestation have also been used to justify abortion. Since the burdens of having children fall only on women and never on men, abortion is justified even if the human fetus is a person. Thomson suggests that it is unjust that *women* have to shoulder this burden of gestation but *men* never have to do so. In a similar vein, Martha Nussbaum points out:

> Under US constitutional law, a heightened level of scrutiny is pertinent for so-called "suspect classifications," those involving groups with a history of discrimination and/or political powerlessness. Race and gender have been two categories so recognized. What this means is that if a law were passed saying that when kidney transplants are needed to save lives (of full-fledged human beings), all and only African Americans must donate their kidneys, this . . . Laws outlawing abortion, many legal scholars argue, are analogous: for they, too, employ a suspect classification, requiring only women to bear the burden of life support for foetuses and thus to jeopardize their own health and opportunities.
>
> (2008, p. 343)

Nussbaum makes a legal point here, but the general argument could also be used to come to an ethical conclusion.

One could attempt to rectify this perceived injustice by requiring that men and women alike must equally come to the aid of others in need, as the Good Samaritan laws of some countries require. However, men cannot, even if they wished to, gestate a child. This alleged unfairness, however, results not from the imposition of power by one group over another as would be the case with forcing all and only African Americans to be organ donors. The disparity that only some women—and not all of them—can get pregnant arises from an intrinsic aspect of the biological reality of humankind. Since mere biological realities can never be "just" or "unjust," the analogy with African Americans fails.

Second, the demands of morality (or law) with respect to abortion choice should not be unequal with respect to male and female. Males and females are equally required not to intentionally kill innocent human beings; thereby, innocent male and female human beings are equally protected. If the human fetus, male or female, is an innocent person, morality should forbid anyone—regardless of gender—from procuring abortion. Indeed, such an ethical norm (or law) may disproportionately interfere with the liberty of men in so far as most abortionists are male. There should be one standard with respect to killing innocent human beings, including human beings prior to birth, and it is a gender neutral standard.

It is true that the burdens of continuing pregnancy fall upon pregnant women and not men, but it is equally true that the burdens of raising children fall upon those who have children and not the childless. It is not, however, a form of unjust age discrimination to forbid killing children, even though this norm will disproportionately burden persons of child bearing age and never burden anyone prior to child bearing age. It is not a form of unjust discrimination against parents to forbid the killing of children, even though this ban will result in parents having an unequal burden in raising children when compared to those who are not parents.

In addition, common morality does indeed allow an unequal distribution of duties and burdens for the common good—and the defense of children is surely a part of the common good. The wealthy pay a greater share of taxes, both proportionately and in absolute terms, than the moderately well off or the poor. In many countries, young men are required to register for and, if need be, to serve in the military, but older men and women are not so required. As Alexander Pruss points out,

> Being drafted seems pretty clearly at least as great an imposition as being required to continue pregnancy. It typically involves one's life being put under the control of higher officers in respect of just about every small detail, whereas only a few pregnancies require quite as much modification of one's life (cases where bed-rest is required for the length of the pregnancy are similar in this respect, though even

then one is free to decide what activities to engage in while in bed, such as reading, writing, listening to the radio, etc.) The danger to life from the draft can be, depending on the conflict, significantly greater than that from pregnancy. Moreover, in being drafted, one becomes put under the orders of a hierarchy that can, and sometimes does, order one to engage in actions that are highly likely to result in one's being severely wounded, captured and tortured, or killed. (I expect that if I were to have to choose on grounds of self-interest, I'd choose pregnancy over serving in the U.S. army in WWII, though I need to go on second and third hand data in both cases.)

(Pruss 2008)

Since the protection of innocent human persons is a fundamental aspect of the common good, unequal distributions of burden need not be unfair.

Even if pregnancy were an unfair burden, it still would not follow that abortion is morally permissible. It is true that the pregnant woman is supporting her child in utero (recall, the supposition of Thomson's argument that the fetus is a full person, so the use of "child" is not begging any questions in this context), so the argument goes the pregnant woman has no obligation to support the baby she carries. Even so, it still doesn't follow she has a right to kill him or her. In general, from the non-existence of a duty to support a right to kill does not follow. As McMahan notes, "It is hard to believe that it is permissible to kill one's own child in order to avoid the burden of providing the aid one has caused it to need" (2002, p. 398).

Finally, as Francis Beckwith points out:

[T]here are burdens that attend the condition of pregnancy that cannot be shared with the male parent, for they are unique to the female of the human species. But it is not clear how the differences in parental burdens between the sexes justifies abortion. It seems to me that the correct comparison is between the burdens to be borne by the child or its mother, not between the father and the mother, if the decision to abort hangs in the balance. For if we were to think of the burden of an ordinary pregnancy as a harm exclusively borne by the woman . . . and compare it to the harm of death borne exclusively by the unborn child if it is aborted, "the harm avoided by the woman seeking the abortion," writes [Patrick] Lee, "is not comparable with the death caused to the child aborted. (Recall that burden need only involve nine months of pregnancy; the woman can put the child up for adoption.)"

(2007, p. 194)

The relevant comparison in considering burdens is not between the mother and father, but rather between the mother and the unborn human child. When this comparison is considered, when death is set against the burdens of pregnancy, there is almost no one who would prefer getting violently killed to having to endure a pregnancy. The burdens of being violently killed clearly are not equal to the burdens of pregnancy, so it is unfair to make one person endure violent death so as to relieve another person of pregnancy.

Critics have also argued that Thomson overestimates the burden of pregnancy in her use of the violinist analogy, which actually bears little resemblance to the reality of pregnancy. As Rosalind Hursthouse notes in the violinist case:

> I cannot do my job, I cannot go visit my sick mother, I cannot go to my sister's wedding, I cannot go to films, I cannot go swimming, I cannot read (well, perhaps the violinist is a great talker), I cannot have a confidential conversation with anyone and I cannot make love. And all of this for a whole nine months. But the usual pregnancy does not make one bed-ridden, and even when it does, very rarely for nine months; nor is the foetus, even assuming it to be a person, someone whose presence rules out reading, private conversations, and sex.
>
> (1987, p. 203)

A pregnancy does not impose (at least in the vast majority of cases) anything like the burden of the violinist. Indeed, some women report feeling even better than normal both psychologically and physically during pregnancy.

However, one must also factor in the burden of becoming a mother (as opposed to being merely pregnant) as a part of the assessment, and this is perhaps the most significant reason abortion is chosen. Some women simply do not want to become mothers; other women do not want to become mothers again, with this partner, or at this time of life. Since becoming a mother is an incredibly significant change in a woman's practical identity, something over which she should be able to exercise control, abortion is morally permissible or at least not indecent (Little 2003, pp. 320–321).

To address this objection, one must distinguish three aspects of parenthood: a social sense (raising or socializing children after birth), a genetic sense (contributing sperm or eggs for conception), and a gestational sense (carrying a developing human). If the human fetus is already a person, then the pregnant woman is already a mother in two senses, gestationally and, aside from some cases of *in vitro* fertilization, also genetically. So, a pregnant woman is already a mother in at least the genetic and gestational senses of the term. It remains for her to choose whether or not to become a mother in the social sense of the term, when a choice which is made for or against adoption. Thus, abortion does not give a woman the chance to decide not to become a mother, but like infanticide gives the woman the choice not to continue to be a mother in the biological and gestational senses.

If women do indeed have the right not to remain mothers, then it would be fair to assert the same right for fathers. They should be permitted not to remain biological fathers (since like mothers they can already choose to be or not to be social fathers). Once the child is in existence, the only way to cease being a biological father or mother is to kill the child in question. Since men could not exercise the right not to be a biological parent without interfering with the right to bodily integrity of their pregnant partner, it would seem the right not to be a biological parent would have to be exercised sometime after birth. Such a right, if made absolute, would be the revival of the ancient Roman custom whereby the father had the right to take the life of even his adult son or daughter. If one believes that infanticide is wrong, we have strong reason to believe that there is no moral right to end one's biological parenthood. If Thomson's supposition of fetal personhood is correct, a pregnant woman already has the burden of motherhood in some sense (gestational and usually genetic), and abortion is not needed to avoid the burden of social motherhood. What is really at issue is continuing the burdens of gestational motherhood.

Let us suppose for the sake of argument that the burdens of pregnancy are much *greater* than the burdens of being a minimally decent father or mother. Undoubtedly, the burdens of pregnancy are tremendously significant, and although they vary from woman to woman there is no doubt that pregnancy, especially crisis pregnancy, can be the most serious challenge a person may face in life. However, in assessing the burdens before making the choice to abort or give birth, one must weigh not only the burdens of carrying and giving birth to the baby but also the burdens of having an abortion.

Does the burdensomeness of abortion make a difference in determining whether abortion is morally permissible? After all, if it is morally permissible to unplug oneself painlessly, surely it is also permissible to unplug yourself at some cost to yourself (Boonin 2003, p. 241).

However, if one accepts the premise of Thomson's original article, the nature of the burden does make a difference, indeed all the difference, in assessing the morality of abortion. If we consider the case of the violinist, Thomson agrees that if the violinist will fully recover in one hour, then you ought to allow him to remain plugged in, and it would be indecent of you to unplug yourself from him and cause his death since the burden to you is slight (Thomson 1971, pp. 59–60). If we only had to be "plugged in" for ten seconds, and it was utterly painless and in other ways unburdensome, it would clearly be impermissible not to give such aid. However, being plugged into the violinist for nine months *is* a tremendous burden, so you may unplug yourself.

But let's change the violinist analogy slightly. What if you had to endure the nine months burden *regardless* of whether or not you caused the violinist to die? Imagine you must remain plugged into a machine for the next nine months, a machine whose operation can, if you choose, also help the violinist to survive until he overcomes his illness. You must endure a substantial burden either way, so the only choice you really have is whether to help the violinist (with no substantially greater cost to you) or not to help him. To cause the violinist to die in *this case* is to cause gratuitous harm to an innocent person without relieving yourself of a substantial burden, and this is obviously wrong. In other words, if the burden to you of keeping the violinist alive, though great, is not substantially *greater* than the burden you would have to endure if you caused his death, then causing his death is impermissible.

Indeed, such is the case with abortion. That abortion itself is sometimes burdensome is noted even by defenders of abortion. As Boonin notes, "To set the [violinist] analogy straight, then, we must specify that the process of unplugging yourself from the violinist also imposes a variety of costs or risks of costs, and of comparable magnitude" (2003, p. 241). The physical costs of abortion can include (but are not limited to) swelling, vomiting, cramps, sterilization, excessive bleeding, and pain. Of course, like bringing a pregnancy to term, these costs are not endured at all or to the same degree by every woman who has an abortion.

Similarly, the psychological costs of continuing with a pregnancy until live birth are significant and can include mood swings, irritability, low libido, and weepiness. However, the same thing may be said of terminating a pregnancy via abortion. The psychological costs of abortion that many women experience from abortion can be great, as acknowledged also by those who nevertheless defend abortion (Boonin 2003, p. 241).

Of course, if the central thesis of this book (as argued in other sections) is correct, namely that the vast majority of abortions are morally impermissible, the greatest cost endured by women who choose abortion is the moral cost. To do anything morally wrong is to disfigure oneself in a moral sense, and the more serious the wrong chosen, the more serious the disfigurement. After the choice of abortion, many women bear a burden of guilt that is, for some, never terminated.

If the costs or risks of costs to women in both choosing abortion and choosing to give live birth are of a similar magnitude, then women in such situations will, *whatever they choose*, have (and/or risk having) significant burdens. Costs or risks of costs for women with crisis pregnancies are a reality that cannot be avoided by abortion.

But perhaps this analysis has overestimated the costs and risks of abortion. It is indeed extremely difficult to do such a comparison because one has to take into account all the various factors such as certain, likely and possible burdens as well as certain, likely, and possible benefits. The best way to assess such factors and burdens "all things considered" would probably be to compare the actual experiences of the women who have gone through abortion and/or childbirth. Such consideration provides evidence, not only against Thomson's defense of abortion, but against all defenses of abortion arising from a concern for the well-being of women.

Among those who have had abortions, some reported that they were satisfied with what took place and if they had to do it over they would choose abortion again. Other women who have had an abortion deeply regretted their decision. Next, we could consider women, in similar circumstances to those who had abortions, who instead chose to give life. Here there is an interesting asymmetry with the first group because, although many women will say that choosing life was the most difficult choice they have ever made, virtually all are glad that they did not have an abortion, including those who initially wanted abortion. They are satisfied with themselves in this regard and live without regret. Indeed, a study found that after birth, the satisfaction of women who had *twice* been denied abortion with their children was not significantly different from those who had not sought abortion (Dytrych, Matejček, Schüller, Friedman, & Friedman 1975, p. 170). "By and large, the study group mothers did move from initial rejection to ultimate acceptance [of the child]" and some 38% of women in the study even denied ever having sought abortion (Dytrych et al. 1975, p. 170). According to another study, women who bring unwanted children to term on the whole do not manifest mental health problems (Najman, Morrison, Williams, Andersen, & Keeping 1991).

Many women regret and suffer because of their abortions. One study indicated that "women who had had an abortion had a significantly higher relative risk of psychiatric admission compared with women who had delivered for every time period examined" (Reardon 2003, p. 834; Morgan, Evans, Peters, & Currie 1997). In comparison with women who gave birth, women who choose abortion are 3.5 times more likely to die within a year and seven times more likely to commit suicide (Gissler et al. 1996). Abortion is linked with substance abuse, eating disorders, guilt, and self-punishment, as well as a variety of physical complications including cervical injuries, perforated uterus, and cancer (Strahan 2001). Whether causation, correlation, or a bit of both explains these links is a question of great importance.

Even aside from this empirical evidence, the critic of abortion can ask pointed rhetorical questions: What woman mourns the anniversary of her child's birth? But how many women mourn usually in silence on the anniversary of an abortion? What woman looks at her child and says, "If only I had aborted her?" But how many women consider in the quiet of their hearts, "If I hadn't had the abortion . . .?" No group calls itself "Women Exploited by Giving Birth" or "Women Victimized by Giving Life." Yet many groups exist to comfort women hurt by abortion such as "Women Exploited by Abortion" or "Women Victimized by Abortion," organizations with thousands of members. No books are published to console women who gave birth rather than aborted. But how many books are published, from both pro-choice and pro-life perspectives, to help women with post-abortion grief? (A small selection includes *The Healing Choice: Your Guide to Emotional Recovery After an Abortion; The Jericho Plan: Breaking Down the Walls Which Prevent Post-Abortion Healing; No One Told Me I Could Cry: A Teen's Guide to Hope and Healing After Abortion; Experiencing Abortion: A Weaving of Women's Words; Peace After Abortion; A Solitary Sorrow: Finding Healing & Wholeness After Abortion;* and *Do Not Lose Hope: Healing the Wounded Heart of Women Who Have Had Abortions.*) Taking into account such empirical and anecdotal considerations, the choice of abortion is itself of possible serious consequence for the woman.

There are of course scores of books published to help women deal with post-partum depression, but post-partum depression seems importantly different than mourning abortion. First, post-partum depression can hit in situations in which the child has been planned and wanted even prior to conception; but in elective abortion the human being in utero is not wanted. What this suggests is that post-partum depression is not *per se* about the child, but rather is due to other factors such as changes in hormones and lack of social support. The sadness that sometimes follows abortion by contrast seems directly related to the choice to end the life of the human being in utero. Second, it is extremely uncommon for post-partum depression to continue years after the birth of the child, but grief over abortion can extend over decades. Most women celebrate the day of their child's birth year after year. By contrast, the day of the abortion is for many women a time of mourning, loss, and sadness year after year. President Barak Obama has spoken of, "the middle aged feminist who still mourns her abortion" (Obama 2008, p. 51). Post-abortion grief is simply not the same as post-partum depression.

Since both abortion and continuing a crisis pregnancy impose (and/or risk imposing) substantial burdens on the woman, *substantial burdens cannot be avoided*. But if this is true, then the critic of Thomson's argument can point out that aborting a person is causing harm to another for no (overall) substantial gain, even if *only* the well-being of the pregnant women is considered. Costs or risks of costs to pregnant women are a reality that cannot be avoided by abortion, so ending the life of the human being in utero is akin to ending the life of the violinist even though you had to remain plugged into the machine that could save his or her life anyway.

Thomson's argument presupposes that two persons are involved in the situation, so the harms caused to both are relevant to consider. Whether pregnancy should be considered as a "harm" or a prima facie good is debated, but suppose that pregnancy is a harm. If we compare the burdens of pregnancy with harm of death, it is obvious that the greater cost would be suffered by the human fetus (Lee 1996, p. 118). If we had to choose between enduring either the burdens of pregnancy or dying, virtually no one would choose death.

7.8 Does Killing Make a Being "Worse Off"?

In her book *Creation and Abortion: A Study in Moral and Legal Philosophy*, Francis Kamm argues that a mother has no duty to aid the human fetus and that the human being in utero is not made worse off by being killed than it would have been if it had never had that for which it had no right (namely, the mother's aid).

> The fetus cannot obtain the right to remain in the woman's body, and she cannot be obligated not to kill it, simply because ending its support would require that we take away the life that it has only because it received the support. . . . [I]f letting it die is permissible, then . . . sometimes killing it is permissible as well.
>
> (1992, p. 81)

If parents do indeed have duties to their own children in virtue of their biological relationship, as I have argued earlier (section 7.6), then Kamm's argument fails. But what about the claim that killing the human fetus does not make it "worse off"? Is the human being in utero merely deprived of what the fetus had not right to enjoy in the first place?

One strange result of this argument is that abortion would be more difficult to justify in all cases in which *in vitro* fertilization (IVF) is used. In cases of IVF, the human embryo planted in the woman's uterus did indeed have other opportunities for life, namely being implanted in another woman's uterus, perhaps even a woman who would not consider having an abortion. In such cases, if abortion is chosen, the human fetus is made worse off than it would have been if it had never been in that woman's body, for it could have been implanted in another woman's body. Now imagine that a woman is taken by force to a lab, and then a human embryo is involuntarily implanted in her womb and contrast this case with a woman who gets pregnant as the result of normal intercourse. On Kamm's view, abortion following an act of voluntary intercourse would be permissible; but abortion chosen following non-voluntary implantation of an IVF embryo would not be (since the embryo is made worse off relative to the other prospects the embryo had prior to implantation). This is greatly counter-intuitive.

Now, even if the human fetus is a person, and even if it is generally wrong to kill a human person, questions still remain in the case of abortion about circumstances of rape, incest, and threat to the mother's life. The defender of abortion can point to certain cases where, intuitively speaking, abortion seems not only morally permissible but plainly desirable. But what shall be said about abortion in cases of moral catastrophes, such as rape or incest? What about the natural catastrophe in which the mother's life is at risk unless she has an abortion? What about the "hard cases"? They are the subject of the next chapter.

8   Is Abortion Permissible in Hard Cases?

The hard cases of abortion, such as fetal deformity, rape, incest, and life of the mother, deserve careful consideration because many people who are otherwise in favor of protecting human life in utero make exceptions in such cases and because for many people, abortion, in these cases, seems so obviously permissible, perhaps even obligatory. However, it would be a mistake to believe that hard cases exist only for critics of abortion. Defenders of abortion also find some cases, such as sex selection abortion or abortion for other trivial reasons, quite difficult to reconcile with common moral intuitions. This chapter will consider first hard cases for critics of abortion, and second, hard cases for defenders of abortion.

Both defenders of abortion and critics note that hard cases make up only a small percentage of all abortions. There is widespread agreement, for example, that abortion in cases of rape constitute only about 1% of all abortions and also that partial-birth abortions constitute less than 1% of all abortions. Despite Mark Twain's warning about "lies, damn lies, and statistics," there seems to be little reason to doubt such statistics. However, the tiny percentage of "hard cases" does not lessen the significance of such cases for two reasons.

The first is that there are millions of abortions performed every year. In the United States alone, the number of abortions ranges between 1.2 and 1.6 million each year. Worldwide the number of abortions yearly is estimated at about 46 million, and in the United States alone, there have been over 42 million since 1973. So even if only 1% of abortions are of a particular type (partial birth or for rape), it still follows that in the United States alone this would be more than 10,000 abortions per year, nearly half a million throughout the world. These are not insignificant numbers.

Furthermore, even if any given kind of abortion took place only a handful of times per year, these abortions still make a gigantic difference for those involved. It is not a comfort to someone dying from a lethal disease that the disease is extremely rare. Though cases of crucifixion and lynching are rare, their rarity makes them no less wrong when they do happen. So for critics of abortion and defenders of abortion alike, the fact that a certain kind of abortion is rare, even extremely rare, makes no important difference to its moral permissibility or impermissibility.

8.1 Hard Cases for Critics of Abortion

8.1.1 Difficult Circumstances

The most common reason for abortion is not rape, incest, or concern for the life of the mother. In fact, these reasons are involved in only a tiny fraction of all abortions. The most common reason for seeking an abortion is simply that the circumstances of the pregnancy are not felt to be right, not right for the mother and not right for the one to be born. Of course, it is impossible to list all the particular circumstances involved in each situation. However, even a partial list of the circumstances present in many cases would include formidable difficulties like: broken families; drug abuse; crushing poverty; abusive relationships; incomplete education; fear of public humiliation; antagonistic partners; failed love. All of these troubles and more are present in many cases.

It would be both arrogant and foolhardy to sit in judgment of women in such circumstances and declare them to be morally inferior because they see abortion as the only way out of a dire predicament. As noted in the introduction, unless one knows the understanding and intention of the person involved, a definitive moral judgment of an agent's moral culpability should never be made, even if at the same time a moral judgment about an agent's actions objectively considered can be made. Indeed, supporting women who find themselves in a dire crisis because of a pregnancy, or indeed for any other cause, is a duty of all people of goodwill regardless of their opinions on abortion. Both critics and defenders of abortion alike characteristically agree on this much.

It is also important to note that all of the circumstances listed above (abuse, poverty, humiliation, etc.) can equally, or even to a greater extent, afflict parents of children after birth. Here too we can find common ground. Both critics and defenders of abortion (and infanticide) would agree that even the most dreadful circumstances would not justify intentionally killing a 6-year-old child. In such a case, both would agree that what must be done is to search zealously for solutions to the problems facing mother and child. Support and love for the woman includes supporting and loving her enough to aid her in doing good, not in doing evil. If something is morally wrong, then it is not truly loving and supportive to aid someone in doing wrong, even if that is what the agent desires to do, at least at the moment. Common morality holds that, intentionally killing an innocent person, or helping others to do so are not ethically permissible solutions, even in dire circumstances. Even if solutions to such problems are not entirely adequate, or cannot be found at all, it still would not be permissible to kill a 6-year-old child intentionally.

Doing what is right or avoiding what is wrong is not always easy. Indeed, in some circumstances, doing what is right or avoiding what is wrong can mean doing what is incredibly difficult, requiring heroic courage. In circumstances like the dire ones described above, both the critic of abortion and defender of abortion would agree that, insofar as we are able, we must aid both mother and child. If there is a human problem, we should seek to eliminate the problem, not eliminate the human.

Where the critic and defender of abortion disagree is, of course, about the status of the human being in utero. But the personhood of the fetus does not depend in any way on whether he or she was conceived within a great family or a lousy one, in a rich woman or in a poor one, in a time of great opportunity or in a time of dashed hopes. You are who you are regardless of the circumstances of your conception and birth. So the argument from dire circumstances does not undermine the personhood of the human embryo, fetus, or newborn. Pointing out that abortion will undermine the economic or sexual well-being of women (Sherwin 1996) would suggest a *prima facie* right to abortion if these harmful side effects were the only consideration. But as Warren writes:

> It is, at best, morally problematic to allow human beings who have a right to life to be killed simply to prevent bad consequences to other human beings. Surely no one is entitled deliberately to kill an innocent human being who has done nothing to waive and forfeit his or her right to life.
>
> (1998, p. 129)

If the human fetus is not a person, dire circumstances would probably not be needed to justify abortion. However, if the fetus is accorded an intermediary moral status as discussed below (8.3.8), perhaps some abortions would be impermissible. However, if the human fetus is a person as much as any 6-year-old, dire circumstances do not justify the termination of his or her life.

8.1.2 Fetal Deformity

The same reasoning applies to cases of fetal deformity. Learning of fetal deformity breaks the hearts of those involved. Perhaps the child was wanted, perhaps conceived only after years of effort. Now, the human being in utero, maybe even already named, turns out to have Down's syndrome, or an even more serious mental or physical handicap. Abortion in such cases is sometimes argued to be for the child's own good.

However, learning of the mental or physical handicap of a child after birth would be no less traumatic, indeed perhaps even more traumatic. At least before birth, normally physicians must run a series of tests to attempt to confirm fetal deformity, giving parents some time to adjust before knowing with certainty that their fears have been realized. After birth, the existence of a perhaps previously unknown deformity could be inescapably evident. It is also clearly true that some people become mentally or physically disabled much later in life, during, for example, their early twenties, when their personhood has been uncontroversially established. The importance of determining when personhood begins is again evident. One could hold that disabled human beings, whether physically and/or mentally disabled, are not persons, so that the human fetus with a serious mental or physical disability is also not a person. Few people, however, believe that disabled adults or school age children with disabilities are not persons. Indeed, most people are horrified to learn of the abuse of the disabled that sometimes takes place. Arguments that would seek to establish the claim that disabled adults are not persons are similar to the arguments already discussed in the first four chapters. By definition, disabled human beings have impaired physical and/or mental function, and so arguments already discussed which deny the personhood of the human fetus might also be used to deny the personhood of an adult human being with a handicap. (This was, for instance, the case with the arguments examined in section 3.6).

Such arguments conceive of personhood in a functional and not ontological way, and so they would be subject to all the criticisms already made of functional conceptions of personhood. Now, if mentally or physically disabled adults and school age children are persons, or if every human being is a person, then mentally or physically disabled human beings in utero would not simply on account of their disability fail to be persons. So aborting a human fetus because he or she is disabled is not substantially different from aborting a human fetus for other reasons. The trauma for parents learning of the fetal deformity cannot be denied, and parents in such a situation need all the comfort, love, and support possible. But since the trauma in question does not justify killing a child after birth, it does not justify abortion before birth either, unless of course birth marks the moment when a human being becomes a person—which, as we saw in chapter three, it does not. Indeed, many people who work or live with the disabled profess that caring for handicapped human beings greatly enriches the human experience (MacIntyre 1999, pp. 138–139).

An especially difficult case involves prenatal diagnosis of diseases known to be fatal shortly after birth. This is a difficult case to handle for the pro-life position because the baby is doomed to death even if abortion is not performed. At least if abortion is performed, the mother is spared continuing with the pregnancy, spared giving birth, and spared the trauma of waiting for the newborn to die. On the principle that we should salvage the best out of even difficult situations such as this, it would seem justifiable to abort the human fetus with a fatal disease so as to spare the mother the trauma that she would have to endure in forgoing abortion.

In considering the ethics of such cases, it is important to note that abortion itself imposes considerable burdens on the woman (section 7.7). Either of the choices available under these horrific circumstances (abortion or allowing the baby a natural death) is likely to be traumatic. With this said, and in view of the dignity of the one who would be aborted, it seems clear that the expectant lifespan of a person does not make a difference in whether or not a person may be killed. The fact that a person at the end of life may have only a short time to live does not imply the permissibility of killing that person. If someone is scheduled to be executed, that fact does not authorize private persons to kill the death row inmate earlier. Indeed, the prospective lifespan of a human person varies a great deal depending upon cultural factors, the race and gender of the person, and the health care available. The prospective lifespan of a human being is irrelevant to the question of the permissibility of killing. So, if the human being in utero is a person, then killing is impermissible even if the human being will die of other causes in a few weeks.

8.1.3 Abortion for the Child's Good

Situations in which the child would be born into dire circumstances or with physical or mental disability are also sometimes said to justify abortion on the grounds that it is in the child's best interest. Such consequentialism depends upon an evaluation of what the child's life will be like in the distant future, for, of course, if you knew that the child would have a wonderful life in the future, then it would not be the case that aborting him or her is in his or her best interest. A judgment that the child's life will not be worth living depends upon an estimation of what his or her future holds.

But is this sort of knowledge even remotely possible? Aside from very rare cases, such as Tay-Sachs, the answer must be "no." Even though you surely know more about yourself than any other person, it is likely that you will find many questions about yourself impossible to answer. Will you be flourishing in 20 years? Will you be absolutely miserable? Perhaps painful illness will overtake you; perhaps future technology will grant you perfect health. Perhaps you will be reduced to begging; perhaps you will be the next Bill Gates. Perhaps you will be hated and infamous; perhaps you will be widely loved and honored. I cannot say what my future holds despite knowing a great deal about my own past achievements and failures, my talents and weaknesses, my joys and frustrations. Knowing yourself as well as you do, I doubt your position differs significantly from mine. But since we don't even know if our own future will be overwhelmingly positive or bitterly negative (or what mixture of each), it is even more difficult to know the future for any given child whose inclinations, desires, talents, and possibilities we simply cannot begin to estimate.

Consider the situation of a father suffering from syphilis and his wife enduring tuberculosis. She finds out that she is pregnant with their fifth child. Of the other children, the first is blind, the second died, the third is deaf, and the fourth also has tuberculosis. Abortion could seem to some as almost a duty in light of such circumstances. Imagine further that the mother has a crystal ball through which she can see some but not all of the future. She finds out that her son, if born, will grow up in adverse circumstances, will endure serious depression, will deeply love someone who does not return his love, and eventually will become entirely deaf, an especially difficult burden due to his passion and profession as a musician.

The son described in the previous paragraph is Ludwig van Beethoven. Of course, there is only one Beethoven, and geniuses of his rank are rare. The point is not simply that abortion is wrong because one might abort a future genius who makes irreplaceable contributions to humanity (although any given abortion may indeed abort a future genius or a future villain). Intentionally inflicting an actual, present, and greater harm, such as taking someone's life, cannot be justified in order to prevent possible, future, and lesser harms.

But is abortion characteristically done to prevent future possible harms to the child or is it rather self-concern that typically motivates the termination of pregnancy? Naomi Wolf doubts whether a consideration of the well-being of the child involved actually motivates most abortions:

> Not to judge other men and women without judging myself, I know this assertion [namely, abortion is undertaken for the child's best interest] to be false from my own experience. . . . If I had been thinking only or even primarily about the baby's life, I would have had to decide to bring the pregnancy, had there been one, to term. No: there were two columns in my mind "Me" and "Baby" and the first won out. And what was in it looked something like this: unwelcome intensity in the relationship with the father; desire to continue to "develop as a person" before "real" parenthood; wish to encounter my eventual life partner without the off-putting encumbrance of a child; resistance to curtailing the nature of the time remaining to me in Europe. Essentially, this column came down to: I am not done being responsive only to myself yet. At even the possibility that the cosmos was calling my name, I cowered and stepped aside. I was not so unlike those young louts who father children and run from the specter of responsibility. Except that my refusal to be involved with this potential creature was as definitive as a refusal can be.
>
> (Wolf 1995, p. 32)

Naomi Wolf seems to view her experience as not exceptional or unique to her, but rather as typical of the reality of what women experience in choosing abortion. To portray the typical abortion as a selfless choice undertaken for the good of the baby is, to use Wolf's phrase, "non-sense."

Even if it were granted that noble motives underlie the choice of abortion in some cases, such motivations still would not change the ethics of the act itself. The motives of an action are ethically relevant in determining whether or not the action as a whole (the act itself, motivation, and circumstances) is morally acceptable. But benevolent motivations cannot justify acts that are in themselves evil and unjust. So, if the argument of the previous chapters has been correct, even if abortion were chosen for the most benevolent of motives, even in cases of Tay-Sachs, the act of abortion itself would still be morally wrong. Disabled human beings— whether they are newborns (as discussed in section 2.5) or human beings in utero—have the same basic moral worth as human beings that are not disabled.

8.1.4 Cases of Rape and Incest

Accordingly, let us now consider abortion in cases of rape and incest, where justification is sought not in an appeal to the good of the child involved but rather in an appeal to the good of the mother. This will allow us to assess the propriety of self-interested motives in their most sympathetically compelling instances. Where incest takes place without informed consent, as it characteristically does, it too is really a form of rape and thus will be treated as such in our discussion.

Even though conception in the case of rape is relatively rare and even though conception can be prevented if the victim receives prompt medical attention (a practice acceptable even to those who oppose contraception, see Finnis 1991, p. 39), nevertheless it turns out that most women who actually conceive a child by rape do not choose to have an abortion. Most give birth and then place the child for adoption; others decide that they themselves will raise the child. Such women transform a horrendously evil act into an opportunity for heroic generosity and service to others. Nevertheless, consider a case in which a woman does want to have an abortion.

As is clear from our discussion thus far, much of the abortion debate revolves around the question of personhood. One way to justify abortion in the case of rape is to say that a human fetus conceived by rape is not a person. However, as we have seen, the circumstances of one's conception, even if conception takes place because of rape, do not seem to make any difference in terms of personhood. Indeed, it could have turned out that you were conceived from an act of rape, but of course, you would still in that case be as much a person were you conceived by consensual intercourse. Even if you were not conceived from an act of rape, it is undoubtedly true that there are many human beings around who are incontrovertibly persons who were conceived through an act of rape—perhaps your best friend, your aunt, or your teacher. Such human beings clearly exist and are undoubtedly persons. So if a human being is conceived from an act of rape, it does not follow that the human being is not a person. Therefore, even if a human fetus is conceived as the result of rape, it does not follow that the human fetus is not a person.

Obviously pregnancy due to rape is horrendously difficult. The just rage felt by those who have been sexually assaulted needs to be fittingly discharged. But is abortion a proper outlet? Abortion cannot undo what has been done in a rape. Abortion doesn't even punish the rapist for what he did. Instead it harms an innocent human being, and, given the health and psychological risks involved in abortion described in chapter seven, puts the woman again in harm's way.

Unfortunately, nothing, including having an abortion, can undo a rape. However, to bear a child conceived in these most difficult of circumstances is to perform an act that is in complete contradiction of what takes place in a rape. In rape, a man assaults an innocent human being; in nurturing life, a woman protects an innocent human being. In rape, a man undermines the freedom of another; in nurturing life, a woman grants freedom to another. In rape, a man imposes himself to the great detriment of another; in nurturing life, a woman makes a gift of herself to the great benefit of another. While, unfortunately, rape once perpetrated can never be undone, the rationalizations, maxims, and motives of rape are never so completely rejected as when someone chooses life in the most difficult circumstances, circumstances that make such a choice heroic. Like other women in crisis situations, women who face pregnancies due to rape deserve unconditional love and compassion whether they choose abortion or not. But true love and compassion includes honesty about difficult moral truths and even, sometimes, a call to heroic generosity.

It may be objected that a morally decent person surely does not need to perform heroic acts, and it is undoubtedly true that someone who brings to term a child caused by rape performs a heroic act. As Thomson notes in an argument explored at greater length in the previous chapter, a Minimally Decent Samaritan differs from a Good Samaritan precisely in not choosing the supererogatory, not choosing to go above and beyond the call of duty. Indeed, there are important moral differences among the morally wrong, the morally permissible, and the morally heroic as Thomson's argument presupposes. Normally, one has a choice between what is morally wrong, what is morally permissible, and what is morally heroic. If I encounter a person soliciting donations for pediatric AIDS, I could steal from her, I could give nothing, or I could give a generous donation.

What Thomson's argument seems to ignore is that some circumstances, including those created by the evil choices of others, can sometimes remove the category of the merely permissible, leaving us with a choice between the morally wrong and the morally heroic. If a dictator orders you to torture your mother to death or face a firing squad, you will be faced with the choice between the morally wrong and the morally heroic. A merely permissible option is not available. In the *Crito* and in the *Apology*, Plato depicts Socrates thrust by the decision of the Athenian jury into a choice between doing evil and suffering evil, a choice between the morally wrong and the morally heroic. Should Socrates escape from prison to avoid an unjust death sentence or should he suffer death rather than do what he believes is wrong? The weight of philosophical discussion from Plato through Kant up to such twentieth-century writers as Dietrich Bonhoeffer urges us to do good and avoid doing evil, even when the personal cost is great, even if we are forced to choose between the morally impermissible and the morally heroic in cases where the merely permissible is not available due to the evil choices of others.

8.1.5 Abortion to Save the Mother's Life

Like pregnancy from rape, dangers to maternal health and life during pregnancy also, for obvious reasons, present tremendously difficult situations. I will focus here on situations in which the life of the mother is threatened, the most difficult case for critics of abortion. If one accepts that all human beings are equal persons, then how does one handle cases in which the life of the mother is in danger? Obviously, this is a most serious situation, especially for those who affirm fundamental human equality. These cases, thanks to contemporary technology, are extremely rare but nevertheless they do happen and so they cannot be simply ignored. There are a number of situations in which abortion would seem to be the only possible way to save the life of the mother. How would an advocate for defense of fetal human life respond?

One possible way is to appeal to a right to self-defense. It can happen that an attacker is morally innocent and yet poses a grave danger to others. Such persons are sometimes called material aggressors. Perhaps, the attacker himself was injected with PCP secretly by another and is now on a homicidal rampage. Perhaps the attacker is mentally deranged and believes that you are trying to kill him. In such cases, it would be permissible for you to kill him in self-defense if there is no other way to save your life. Cases of pregnancy in which a human fetus endangers the life of the mother might be analyzed in a similar way. Obviously, the human fetus is not voluntarily and intentionally attempting to kill the mother, but nevertheless a human fetus might be considered a material aggressor. In other words, a lethal threat to the mother is caused by the human fetus, although obviously not intentionally caused by the human being in utero. If lethal self-defense is permissible against material aggressors, and if the human fetus in such circumstances is a material aggressor, then abortion to save the life of the mother is morally permissible (Donagan 1977).

Another way to approach such cases would be through double-effect reasoning (DER). Double-effect reasoning, sometimes also called the doctrine of double effect or the principle of double effect, treats cases in which one act has two effects, one good but the other bad. Double-effect reasoning is used to analyze many moral situations having nothing whatsoever to do with abortion—including physician assisted suicide, bombing a military target when civilians will be killed as a side effect, and administration of drugs with harmful side effects. Although various formulations have been given dating back at least to the thirteenth century, Thomas Cavanaugh has summarized DER in the following way: performing an act with two morally significant effects is justified if (1) the evil effect is not intended as a means or an end, and (2) there is a proportionately serious reason for allowing the evil effect (Cavanaugh 1996). A bit was said in the previous chapter about the importance of the intention/foresight distinction (section 7.4.4), so now a word is in order about the second condition.

Some people object to DER on the basis that "it is pernicious, since it allows the agent to do bad things (all things considered) as long as his intentions are pure" (Harris and Holm 2003, p. 114). This objection rests on a misunderstanding of DER. If we return to the example of the dentist, who fully foresees that she will cause pain but does not intend to cause pain, it may still be the case that inflicting pain is impermissible. Even if the dentist in question is only foreseeing that torturous pain will be caused by a procedure, this is not enough to justify the act if there is not a proportionately serious reason for allowing the pain. Let's take the case of parents considering a dental procedure for their child. The dentist explains that the pain caused by this procedure is extremely severe and cannot be relieved and the good benefit sought by the procedure is merely cosmetic, for example, to increase slightly the whiteness of one tooth in the back of the child's mouth. In such a case, there is not a proportionate reason for allowing the evil effect of torturous pain, even though the evil effect is not intended by the dentist, and so the parents would do wrong if they authorized such a procedure for their child, and the dentist would do wrong if they performed it. On the other hand, if such torturous pain were a side effect of a life-saving intervention, then there would be a proportionately serious reason for the procedure. DER only permits an act with two effects if the evil effect is neither a means nor an end and if there is a proportionately serious reason for allowing the evil effect. Only if both conditions are met is the act in question morally permissible. So it is simply not the case that DER allows an agent to do bad things, all things considered, if his or her intentions are good.

If we apply DER to cases of abortion, the first condition of DER will help us properly distinguish abortion as direct or indirect. It is important to draw a distinction between abortion where fetal death is intentionally brought about (sometimes called "direct abortion") and procedures in which the death of the human being in utero is not intentionally brought about but is a side effect of what a person does intentionally bring about (sometimes called "indirect abortion"). Direct abortion is properly defined as the intentional killing of the human fetus, that is, killing a human fetus either as a means or as an end. Thus, direct abortion would not be permissible according to DER, since DER excludes intending an evil effect (the death of an innocent person) as a means or as an end. Indirect abortions on the other hand would include all acts which bring about the death of the human fetus but in which the agent is not seeking the death of the fetus as an end or as a means. Fetal death is in such cases a side effect, and in accord with the principles of DER may be acceptable for a proportionately serious reason.

Among those who affirm the fundamental equality of all human beings, there is widespread acceptance of the idea that some abortions are indirect and justified. There is, however, no such firm agreement about how precisely to parse the distinction between intention and foresight, and so this leads to some disagreement about which cases of fetal death are direct abortion and which cases of fetal death are indirect abortion. However, there is also widespread agreement about the nature of a proportionately serious reason for causing a foreseen but unintended death. As Bernard Nathanson argues:

> In morality, life can only be equated with life, not with convenience or sociology or politics or economics or poverty . . . In arguing an issue of life, one can only invoke issues of life to counterbalance it.
> (Nathanson 1979, p. 240)

Saving the life of the mother is a proportionately serious reason for allowing a human being in utero to die. Even the staunchest critics of abortion accept this proposition.

Let us consider three cases in which the life of the mother can be at risk: ectopic pregnancy, a pregnant woman with uterine cancer, and a case where the baby has trouble exiting the birth canal.

In ectopic pregnancy, the human embryo does not implant in the uterus but rather elsewhere in the woman's body, often in the fallopian tube. The frequency of ectopic pregnancy has increased some 600% in the last two decades (Diamond 1999, p. 5). When the human embryo implants in the fallopian tube (or even more rarely, elsewhere), the pathology can lead to profuse bleeding and loss of both maternal and embryonic human life. Ectopic pregnancy may be treated in five different ways, including salpingectomy (removal of tube with embryo), salpingostomy (removal of embryo alone), and by use of methotrexate (MXT). Although there is ongoing discussion of treatment options, especially the use of methotrexate, each of these options has been defended as permissible in accord with double-effect reasoning by scholars who accept that every human being is a person.

In the past, doctors regularly used salpingectomy, the removal of the entire fallopian tube with the embryo inside it, to treat ectopic pregnancy. At later stages of ectopic pregnancy, when the fallopian tube has already been badly damaged, salpingectomy is still medically indicated.

In the 1940s, T. L. Bouscaren suggested that salpingectomy is acceptable for those who view the human embryo as a person because the tube itself is pathological and its removal justified by double-effect reasoning (DER). Although the embryonic human life within the tube will die, the surgeon does not intend the embryo's death but only foresees it has a side effect of removing the tube that threatens the woman's life. Almost all critics of abortion accept the permissibility of this practice. The removal of the embryo alone may also be acceptable according to DER, if the removal of the embryo is not considered killing the embryo intentionally. Reported cases of successful implantation of such embryos in utero suggest that removing the embryo from the tube is not always equivalent to killing the embryo (Shettles 1990). Others who affirm the equality of all human beings have argued that using methotrexate, a drug which inhibits rapidly dividing cells such as the early embryo and trophoblast, does not violate DER (Moraczewski 1996a, 1996b); others have challenged this view (May 1998). In sum, there are a number of ways to treat ectopic pregnancy, some or perhaps even all of which do not involve direct abortion. I have explored the ethics of these interventions at greater length elsewhere (Kaczor 2009).

In what has come to be called "the hysterectomy case," a woman is diagnosed with aggressive uterine cancer. Coincidentally, she is also pregnant and, at this stage in pregnancy, the prenatal human being is not yet viable. If the doctor waits to remove the uterus (hysterectomy) until the child is viable, the aggressive cancer will assuredly lead to the woman's death. If the doctor does not wait to remove the uterus, and instead removes it immediately, then the woman will survive but the child will certainly die. Does she commit suicide, if she chooses not to have her uterus removed? Does she have an abortion, if she chooses to remove her uterus knowing that her progeny is not yet viable?

Neither, actually. She may decide that she does not want to have a hysterectomy although she foresees that this choice will allow the cancer to spread and eventually take her life. Perhaps she has cancer in other parts of her body, and perhaps this is her first child. In such a situation, she may want to help another person continue to live rather than add just a few months to her own life at the cost of ending the life within. On the other hand, she might rightfully defend her own life, foreseeing but not intending the death of the developing human within her that will result from the hysterectomy. Neither choice is for death as a means or as an end, but both choices are for life: either for her own life or for her child's life. If the uterus is removed, the death of the human being in utero is not chosen as a means or as an end but is accepted for the proportionately serious reason of preserving the mother's life. If the uterus is not removed, the death of the mother is not chosen as a means or as an end but is accepted for the proportionately serious reason of preserving the life of the human being in utero. Neither choice involves directly killing an innocent human being; both choices are morally permissible.

In what has come to be called "the craniotomy case," a different problem exists. Though virtually always detected before delivery in developed nations, cephalo-pelvic disproportion can result in a situation in which a woman and child may die during an attempted delivery. The child's head is simply too large to pass through the birth canal. The alternatives are stark. It would seem that either the doctor does nothing and both mother and child perish or the doctor crushes the child's skull killing the child and facilitating an end to the labor. If the doctor does nothing, four outcomes are possible. First, both mother and child may die in the course of labor. Second, the baby may die in the course of labor, thereby rendering entirely unproblematic the crushing of the skull ending the labor and preserving the mother's life. Third, it may happen that the mother dies in the course of labor, in which case the child may be safely removed by cutting open the corpse. Finally, both mother and child may live if the child's head narrows and mother's birth canal distends enough to overcome the initial cephalo-pelvic disproportion. On the other hand, the doctor may intervene by crushing the head of the child, thereby both ending the life-threatening delivery and killing the child so that the mother may live. In the craniotomy case, many authors hold that the death of the child is intended.

However, John Finnis, Germain Grisez, Joseph Boyle, and other critics of abortion have noted that in neither the hysterectomy case nor the craniotomy case does the death of the child, as a means or as an end, secure the life of the mother (Finnis et al. 2001, pp. 21–30). Indeed, they defend what is sometimes called a "narrow" view of intention in a series of other cases as well. According to this view of intention, the death is merely foreseen and not intended because the physician does not deliberate about how to achieve the death of the child nor does seeking the death of the child constrain the doctor's other intentions. Unlike a partial-birth abortion, the doctor does not endeavor to achieve the death of the child, and were the death not to come about, it would not be considered a failure of either the proximate or remote ends planned by the doctor. Thus, if a narrow account of intention is used, the death of the child in the craniotomy case need not count as intended.

However, even with this view of intention, one could still argue that craniotomy is morally prohibited by maintaining that it is the crushing of the skull that is wrong and not merely the death of the child. Donald Marquis notes a weakness in the strategy, a weakness that threatens to undermine the distinction on which double-effect reasoning relies:

> The difficulty with this strategy is that if we ask why crushing the child's skull is morally wrong, the answer surely is that it causes the death of the child. If the child's skull could be crushed without irreparable harm or death to the child and the child could be removed from the mother's birth canal thereby saving the mother's life, it is hard to believe anyone would want to condemn the action. Hence, strictly speaking, crushing the child's skull is in itself wrong only because the action can, as a matter of fact, be redescribed as killing the child. But, of course, we can describe the hysterectomy . . . in the same way.
>
> (Marquis 1991, p. 523)

There may be, however, an option that both preserves the account of intention described here and also excludes the craniotomy case. Even if crushing the head of a child is not killing as a means to saving the mother, it may involve another evil means, namely the mutilation or violation of the physical integrity of the child. Were this to be true, we could distinguish the craniotomy case and hysterectomy case and yet retain the insight that the craniotomy case is not killing as a means to saving the mother. But is it mutilation? And is this mutilation nothing other than killing, as Marquis assumes?

Violating the physical integrity of a person, sometimes called mutilation, might be defined as the intentional destruction or removal of an organ (or other body part) that inhibits the function that the organ (or body part) had in maintaining the health of the one possessing the organ. Hence, removal of a diseased or threatening organ is not mutilation because the organ either no longer contributes to the good of the body or threatens no longer to contribute to the good of the body. Nor is removal of superfluous or duplicated organs mutilation because this removal does not inhibit the function that such organs may have had in maintaining health. Thus, kidney donation is licit because removal of a single kidney does not inhibit the function that the kidney once had in the body of purifying the blood supply.

Now, in the craniotomy case, the crushing of the skull, along with the removal of the brain, destroys the functioning of the skull in protecting the brain and thereby damages the most important organ of a well-developed human person. This mutilation does indeed lead to death, as does the removal of other organs without due replacement, such as the liver or heart; but mutilation in itself is not defined in terms of this consequence. Thus, removal of two healthy eyes is mutilation, even though it does not lead to death. Is craniotomy intentional mutilation? Is intentionally violating someone's physical integrity always wrong, even if another will die as a result of non-mutilation? An answer to these questions depends, of course, on how precisely one distinguishes intention and foresight and on how one defines the wrongfulness of mutilation, both matters of great importance and of great difficulty, but matters which I will leave here as open questions.

There are, of course, other cases besides ectopic pregnancy, uterine cancer, and cephalo-pelvic disproportion in which the life of the mother can be threatened by pregnancy (Nathanson 1979, pp. 245–247). However there are no cases where the actual *death* of the child is needed to secure the well-being of the mother, as either a means or an end. Unlike the case of killing to get an inheritance or killing because you hate the person or killing to avoid the responsibility of caring for a person, cases which pit the mother's life against the child's life could be considered indirect abortion so long as the child's death is sought neither as a means nor as an end, but merely accepted as a side effect of a procedure that secures the mother's well-being. Indeed, intending the death of the child sometimes brings greater risk to the life of the mother. For example, in a partial-birth abortion, the human fetus must be inverted and surgical instruments inserted in the birth canal. Both these procedures can pose risks to maternal health not present in normal vaginal birth. In saline injection abortions, women have died when the injection missed its mark. In sum, even the most ardent critics of abortion admit the permissibility of "indirect" abortions aimed at saving the life of the mother. Since saving a person's life is a proportionately serious reason for allowing an innocent person to die, indirect abortion in such circumstances is fully justified.

8.2 Cases of Conscience

Defenders of abortion and critics of abortion sometimes also disagree about the role of conscience. In November 2007, the American College of Obstetricians and Gynecologists (ACOG), Committee on Ethics, issued committee opinion number 385 titled "The Limits of Conscientious Refusal in Reproductive Medicine" (ACOG 2007). The committee enumerates a series of recommendations that "maximize accommodation of an individual's religious or moral beliefs while avoiding imposition of these beliefs on others or interfering with the safe, timely, and financially feasible access to reproductive health care that all women deserve" (ACOG 2007, p. 2). The ACOG appeals to a definition of conscience as "the private, constant, ethically attuned part of the human character." An appeal to conscience would express a sentiment such as, "If I were to do 'x,' I could not live with myself/I would hate myself/I wouldn't be able to sleep at night" (2007, p. 2).

In the ACOG opinion, conscience reflects not one's best judgment at the conclusion of a process of moral deliberation from fundamental moral principles about what is right and wrong all things considered (*ultima facie*), but a feeling that is merely a matter of a provider's personal experience of loss of self-respect. The committee opinion thus construes claims of conscience as *prima facie* values that can and should be "overridden" by the agent in light of other moral considerations (ACOG 2007, p. 3). When this idiosyncratic desire not to feel shame is set against the well-being of a patient, naturally the patient's well-being trumps the private, sentimental desire to keep one's hands clean. The ACOG conception of conscience as a *prima facie* guide contradicts, for example, the proximate supremacy of conscience as an unconditional command (Kant), a magisterial dictate (Newman), and Butler's famous dictum of conscience, "were its might equal to its right, it would rule the world." Sophocles' *Antigone*, Socrates in the *Crito*, and Thomas Aquinas in the *Summa theologiae* (I-II, Q 19.5) all testify that an agent's best ethical judgment—the judgment of conscience—simply cannot be overridden by the agent, if the agent is going to avoid wrongdoing.

In addition, the ACOG recommendations themselves are also highly objectionable. "Physicians and other health care professionals have the duty to refer patients in a timely manner to other providers if they do not feel that they can in conscience provide the standard reproductive services that patients request" (2007, p. 5). This recommendation proposes a duty to cooperate in the wrongdoing of another by helping patients precisely in their wrongdoing. It would indeed be absurd to say, "I would have a guilty conscience if she did 'x.'" (ACOG 2007, p. 2). However, it is not at all absurd to say, "I would have a guilty conscience if I helped her to do 'x.'" Would it really "absolve" a physician from guilt if he did not personally prescribe a drug in order for a patient to commit date rapes, but rather knowingly helped the rapist achieve his goal by referring him to another doctor to fill the prescription?

The ACOG opinion not only unfairly limits a doctor's liberty in action but also infringes upon a physician's freedom of speech. In other contexts, the ACOG has argued against "gag rules" that inhibit a physician from communicating to the patient about what is, in the physician's judgment, relevant for making sure the patient can give informed consent and proper treatment (ACOG 2007, p. 6). However, in opinion 385, physicians may not even communicate their own views about treatment unless they parrot "professionally accepted characterizations of reproductive health services." Such physicians are also forced, even in contexts where such matters may not be at issue, to make their views known to patients, and yet at the same time the new ACOG gag rule forbids them to indicate why they hold these views.

The flawed understanding of conscience accepted by opinion 385 actually commits the ACOG, by extension and analogy, to repugnant positions. The same rules, for example, adopted in a different cultural and legal milieu, would only allow a conscientious objector not to perform female genital mutilation (FGM) so long as the objector was forced to refer patients to those that do perform female genital mutilation. If the physician believes that FGM goes against his or her conception of good medicine, not only must the physician act in certain circumstances against what he or she believes is medically indicated, but the objector must also parrot "professionally accepted characterizations" of the practice, as understood in the predominant cultural and enforced legal milieu without "use of their professional authority to argue or advocate" against FGM. Would such rules, for the physician practicing in places where FGM is legally and culturally accepted, provide an adequate protection (let alone "maximize accommodation") for the doctor conscientiously objecting to FGM? Physicians should not be cast into the role of medical automatons forced to perform actions contrary to their best ethical or medical judgment.

Consider another example. A physician working in a correctional facility is asked to facilitate giving a lethal injection to a prisoner on death row. The physician firmly believes that capital punishment is immoral and further, having closely followed this prisoner's case, is convinced the condemned prisoner is actually innocent. However, let us suppose that state law allows only employees of the correctional facility to be in the room during the execution, and since he is the only physician employed in the prison, according to the principles for conscience set by the ACOG, the physician has a duty to help execute the prisoner. Likewise, in places where euthanasia or physician-assisted suicide is legal, similar conscience guidelines would require physicians opposed to these practices in certain circumstances to kill or help kill their patients. Surely, however, the demands of conscience must not be gerrymandered by the availability of less enlightened and conscientious people.

One of ACOG's concerns is that the exercise of conscientious objection does not create, or reinforce, racial discrimination or socio-economic inequalities in society. However, the ACOG opinion itself creates a professional environment discouraging if not prohibitive to anyone who opposes abortion, for example Catholic and Evangelical Christians who are pro-life. Thus, in its effects, opinion 385 reinforces prejudice and discrimination in the medical profession against both religious minorities and ethnic minorities who are disproportionately Catholic and Evangelical, such as Latinos and African Americans.

8.3 Hard Cases for Defenders of Abortion

8.3.1 *Murder of Pregnant Women*

Hard cases also exist for defenders of abortion. One case that is difficult to reconcile with a denial of the moral status of the preborn is the horror with which we view an assault on a pregnant woman, especially when the assault causes a miscarriage. The murder of a pregnant woman is even more odious and does not seem to be accounted for simply by the consideration that a pregnant woman, like the very young or very old, are vulnerable human persons. Even the most die-hard proponents of capital punishment balk at executing a pregnant woman. Of course, these moral judgments make sense on the supposition that the human being in utero has moral standing, something denied by the standard pro-choice position.

The most typical case of this sort involves either the assault or the murder of a pregnant woman. This may sometimes take place precisely because of the pregnancy. A man tries to convince a woman to have an abortion. She refuses, and he becomes violent. If a pregnant woman is assaulted and loses the pregnancy, should the person be charged with simple assault on her person and nothing more? If a husband murders his pregnant wife, should he be charged with one or two counts of murder? This question became very real when there was debate in California about whether Scott Peterson should have been charged for one or two murders for the slaying of his wife Laci, who was eight months pregnant with their son Conner. Missing since Christmas Eve 2002, their bodies washed up, separately, on shore on April 14, 2003. Conner's umbilical cord was still attached. Despite protest from abortion rights advocates over recognition of Conner's rights, the husband was charged with two counts of murder, with "special circumstances" that allow for tougher penalties. Many states in the United States have similar "fetal homicide" laws. Similar reasoning applies in the assault of a pregnant woman that leads to miscarriage. If the fetus is merely a part of her body, a blob of tissue with less value than a guppy, with no independent moral standing, then she would seem to suffer no important loss (beyond, of course, the important loss constituted by the assault on her person). But if she does suffer a greater loss than is endured by the assault, then this would seem to point to the value of fetal human life. The added horror brought by an assault or murder of a pregnant woman makes sense on the presupposition that the human fetus has moral status, unlike say a guppy or tumor. (Cases of "intermediate" moral status will be discussed below.)

8.3.2 Sex Selection Abortion

Another difficult case for defenders of abortion emerges when abortion is for the purposes of eliminating a human fetus of unwanted gender: sex selection abortion (SSA). Sex selection abortion almost always means the elimination of females, and in some countries is not limited to abortion but extends also to infanticide. Although the preference for males is weaker in predominantly Catholic countries in Central and South America (Warren 1999, p. 139), in the United States, some 85% of women and some 95% of men would prefer to have a male first child. In other countries, especially those in the Far East and Muslim countries, the preference for male children is even stronger. If abortion does not kill a human person, if abortion is, as Warren for instance claims, no more serious than killing a guppy, then abortion of a human because of gender would be permissible. Some abortion defenders might argue that virtually no one would abort simply on the grounds of gender, but, in fact, sex selection abortions and female infanticide take place throughout the world, indeed often in great numbers, particularly in India and China, but also in the United States. Yet if the human fetus has no moral status, then sex selection abortion would seem as permissible as other forms of abortion.

Many feminist defenders of abortion would undoubtedly be troubled by such a conclusion. But how could they consistently criticize sex selection abortions without also implying that abortion in general is problematic? Many pro-choice advocates hold that sex selection abortion is morally problematic, if not impermissible. However, some arguments against SSA only make sense on the implicit assumption that the human fetus is a person with rights, but this premise renders problematic not just SSA but abortion generally. Wishing to avoid this implicit assumption, Wendy Rogers, Angela Ballantyne, and Heather Draper (2007) in their article, "Is Sex-Selective Abortion Morally Justified and Should it Be Prohibited?" provide several arguments that sex selection abortion (SSA) is wrong, without endorsing (they believe even implicitly) the intrinsic value of the human fetus as female or male (Rogers et al. 2007).

Sex selection can occur in three ways, prior to conception via sperm separation, after conception but before implantation via genetic diagnosis of IVF embryos, and after implantation via abortion. In a consideration of sex selection outside of the context of genetically sex-linked diseases, J.M. Milliez notes in his article, "Sex Selection for non-Medical Purposes" that the first

> technique [e.g., sperm separation] raises very few ethical objections. [I]n 2001, the Ethics Committee of the American Society for Reproductive Medicine (ASRM) considered that, in the absence of robust arguments in favor of any potential harm, preconception sex selection was not hazardous and therefore any ban would be unjustified.
>
> (2007, p. 114)

About sex selection after conception via selection and implantation of only male (or female) embryos, much less ethical consensus exists. Some defend it as an exercise of "procreative liberty," but others condemn it as discrimination against gender equality. This sex selection via pre-implantation genetic diagnosis is forbidden by law in India, South Australia, Canada, the United Kingdom, and in ten other European countries.

The third technique of sex selection is most widespread and the most condemned—abortion of the male or female fetus sometime into pregnancy. Detection and eradication of the developing female (or male) fetus can occur quite early in pregnancy.

> A single blood sample is sufficient to recognize the embryo as male or female as early as the first weeks of pregnancy, enabling the elimination of any embryo of undesirable sex with an anti-progesterone medication. However, this method is strictly restricted to the screening of sex-linked genetic disorders or the management of Rhesus immunization. Its use for sex selection for personal convenience is unanimously banned.
>
> (Milliez 2007, p. 115)

In point of fact, abortion for sex selection is not unanimously banned but remains legal in many places, among them the United States and Canada where abortion is officially permitted for any reason. It is true, however, that many people who describe themselves as pro-choice nevertheless oppose sex selection abortion. "Nearly all societies of reproductive medicine, including the American College of Obstetricians and Gynecologists (ACOG 1996), are opposed to sex selection abortion" (Milliez 2007, p. 116). However, from a pro-choice perspective, there is some difficulty in explaining why fetal killing for gender preference should be wrong. Indeed, some of the arguments given for condemnation of SSA would seem equally to apply to sperm separation or pre-implantation selection which is often defended on grounds of reproductive liberty. Other arguments against SSA apply equally to all kinds of abortion. Of course, it is consistent simply to say that any abortion, chosen for any reason including wanting not to give birth to a girl, is ethically permissible, but relatively few people who call themselves pro-choice embrace this consistent position.

Rogers et al. in their article "Is Sex-Selective Abortion Morally Justified and Should it Be Prohibited?" provide several arguments that sex selection abortion (SSA) is wrong, a view many think compatible with a general defense of abortion-choice. They therefore accept the "argument that we should try to understand women's decision to use SSA and empathize with the unjust choice they are forced to make, without accepting that the practice itself is morally justified" (Rogers et al. 2007, p. 522).

The first argument adduced for the conclusion that SSA is wrong is that on either a broad or a narrow interpretation of autonomous choice, SSA practiced in countries with a strong son preference is not an autonomous choice because society puts tremendous pressure on women to have male children, thereby undermining the preferences they would otherwise have.

It is unclear whether Rogers et al. are addressing the objective morality of the act or the subjective responsibility of the agent. I have assumed here that they are addressing the former, since they, as the title of the article suggests, primarily addresses the question of whether SSA is morally justified and should be prohibited. If the point is simply that those who choose SSA in certain contexts are coerced into choices they would rather not have made, then their point is not controversial, or limited to SSA.

SSA is not considered wrong in itself by these authors, but only wrong in the circumstances of a certain cultural context. They simply do not consider the ethics of someone, for example, in Indiana who aborts a boy because of a preference for a girl. What would or would not count as the relevant "cultural context" is similarly not taken up. What if you were from India but now live in Indianapolis? What if you split time between both places and are, by birth and heritage, multi-cultural? It seems odd to hinge the ethics of killing human beings prior to birth because of their gender on cultural context.

Second, the suppressed premise in the argument seems to be that a choice is morally wrong if your autonomous self wouldn't make it. Rogers et al. give no argument for this premise. If the premise were accepted, it would be the case that many abortions as now performed in the United States (not just SSA in India or China) are morally wrong because they are not freely chosen by women but rather only submitted to under pressure from other people.

Rogers et al. also appeal to other considerations in condemning SSA. "A second and separate reason why SSA is morally unjustified relates to the harms that attach to the practice. These include perpetuation of discrimination against women, disruption to social and familial networks, and increased violence against women" (Rogers et al. 2007, p. 522). Milliez also registers this objection to SSA seemingly on behalf of the female fetus herself:

> [E]limination of girls is philosophically and morally unacceptable if perceived as a gender discrimination practice contrary to the principle of equality and in conflict with Kant's moral [teaching] and the notion that all children must be considered as an end, not as a means.
>
> (2007, p. 116)

Likewise, the International Federation of Gynecology and Obstetrics issued a statement, reproduced in Milliez's article, which expressed "concerns about the selection for children with presumed gender characteristics desired by their parents rather than being an end in and of themselves." (Milliez 2007, p. 116). SSA is wrong because it is a form of unjust discrimination.

The question is: Against whom is this unjust discrimination practiced? Given a denial of fetal personhood, the discrimination in question cannot be against the human fetus herself or himself. Discrimination is only problematic when practiced against persons who merit equal and just treatment. To discriminate between non-persons, for example, plucking the red roses, but leaving the white, is not ethically problematic in itself, since these plants do not have rights nor do they merit equal respect as persons. Since the human fetus is not considered a person on the typical pro-choice view, concerns about discrimination against the human fetus should not be relevant in considering actions taken against humans prior to birth.

However, if the male or female fetus is a person, then not just sex selection abortion, but abortion generally becomes problematic. Taken at face value the following quotation from Milliez renders all abortion morally condemnable: "all children must be considered as an end, not as a means" (2007, p. 117). On the other hand, if abortion in general does not end the lives of "girls" and "children" to use Milliez's language, then SSA cannot be problematic on this ground. The pro-choice view generally is that we can accord women the respect they deserve as ends in themselves without extending this respect to female human beings in utero. Obviously, if all human females (and males) merit respect as ends in themselves regardless of age or state of dependence, then not just SSA but all abortion is problematic. On the other hand, if the female fetus is not a person, then presumably one can respect the rights of adult female human beings and nevertheless kill fetal female human beings. Perhaps, the idea is that a sex-selected child, once born and unquestionably a person, will have been treated (when not yet a person) as a mere means to the parents' ends by the selection process. But it is difficult to see why this would be wrong because it is not obviously immoral to treat non-persons as means to one's end. The fact that such non-persons may later be transformed into persons is not relevant to its status at the time of selection.

Rather than appeal to discrimination against the fetus herself, Rogers et al. (2007) ground the wrongness of SSA in terms of its perpetuating discriminatory views such as that girls are worthless burdens whose births should be prevented. As such SSA is viewed as a discriminatory and oppressive practice that fails to accord women the respect they deserve.

Given current cultural milieus, this rationale covers not SSA of males, but only of females. In addition, no developed account is given for the questionable assumption that SSA perpetuates discriminatory views which negatively affect women and girls in society. Indeed, some have suggested that widespread SSA of females prior to birth would seem not to decrease the value of women but rather to increase their perceived value. In the words of Milliez, "[T]he profound gender imbalance [in India and China] has led to a dramatic scarcity of girls who are now regarded as most valuable" (2007, p. 115). Of course, a sound understanding of the human person would not accord value to him or her in terms of being wanted or unwanted by others. Human beings should not be valued according to the laws of supply and demand ("being wanted") as if they were commercial goods, but rather human beings should be valued for their inherent dignity. But if all human beings, regardless of the laws of supply and demand have intrinsic value, then the human fetus also has intrinsic value, a conclusion most defenders of abortion reject.

Finally, Rogers et al. appeal to the bad consequences of SSA:

> A further harm from SSA lies in the resultant severe imbalance in the sex ratio, leading to millions of men being unable to find a partner and found a family. . . . The likely social effects are thought to include increased criminal behavior and social disruption with banditry, violence, and revolutions historically more common in areas with large numbers of excess males.
>
> (2007, p. 522)

I believe that it is correct that SSA as practiced in India and China harms those societies. But the defender of abortion must be careful not to rely too heavily on the premise that SSA is wrong and may be outlawed on this basis. Evidence has been adduced that abortion generally is harmful to society: psychologically, physically, and socially harmful to the women who undergo them (Strahan 2001), and harmful to the culture that allows its weakest and most vulnerable members to be terminated by private force (Spitzer 2000). If this evidence is correct, not just SSA but also abortion in general undermines the common good.

However, some defenders of abortion appeal to the good of society in justifying abortion, arguing that abortion reduces population and thereby promotes the common good. Given these assumptions, SSA of females would be particularly good for society, since a disproportionate reduction in females limits population much more effectively that an equal reduction of male and female. One male can father virtually limitless numbers of children, but each woman can only bear relatively few. Women are the limiting factor in reproduction. Since one man can father more children in a month than any woman could bear in an entire lifetime, the most effective way to reduce population is to reduce the number of females.

A final reason given to oppose SSA is that it leads to an increase in violence against women. Rogers et al. admit that this connection is based on merely anecdotal evidence. However, even if SSA does increase the likelihood of violence against women, evidence has also been given that abortion generally is connected with increased violence against women (Strahan 2001). Thus, the rationale given to condemn SSA may apply equally to abortion undertaken for other reasons.

Many of these consequences would arise equally from the non-existence of adult women from the other forms of sex selection such as sperm separation or implantation of IVF embryos of the desired sex. If aborting a female perpetuates discriminatory views about women, why would sperm selection in order to preclude conception of a female be any different? If disruption of gender balance alone is decisive for condemnation of SSA, why does it matter if this imbalance arises because of sperm separation or SSA? As noted earlier, many individuals and groups hold that sex selection prior to conception is morally unproblematic, but the societal ills recognized by Rogers, Ballantyne, and Draper and others obtain equally whether the gender imbalance takes places through SSA or through sperm separation. It is not a simple matter to condemn SSA while upholding abortion for other reasons.

8.3.3 Abortion for Frivolous Reasons

Another case that would seem to give pause to many advocates of abortion is where abortion is executed for frivolous reasons, such as to eliminate fetuses with undesired traits. Perhaps parents desire a child of above average height, or blue eyes, or athleticism. After amniocentesis, if the human fetus does not have moral status, then abortion chosen because the child has genetic dispositions to be a short, brown-eyed klutz would not be morally impermissible. Imagine a devoted follower of astrological predictions who believes strongly that all relationships with people born under the astrological sign of Leo, sexual or otherwise, are doomed to failure. Then, the doctor makes the terrible announcement that the baby is due in early August. Would abortion to avoid a Leo be permissible? Naomi Wolf notes that some abortions are in fact undertaken for very frivolous reasons:

> Of the abortions I know of, these were some of the reasons: to find out if the woman could get pregnant; to force a boy or man to take a relationship more seriously; and, again and again, to enact a rite of passage for affluent teenage girls. In my high school, the abortion drama was used to test a boyfriend's character. Seeing if he would accompany the girl to the operation or, better yet, come up with the money for the abortion could almost have been the 1970s Bay Area equivalent of the 50s fraternity pin.
>
> (1995, p. 32)

Abortion to add drama to a relationship by seeing how a boyfriend will react seems morally problematic, but the defender of abortion cannot say why, if indeed the human fetus is of no more moral worth than a guppy, and the rights of actual persons always take precedence over "potential" persons.

8.3.4 Safe and Legal, but Why Rare?

Even some ardent defenders of abortion will sometimes affirm that they want abortion to be safe, legal, and rare, but explaining why they should want fewer abortions proves difficult. If nothing is wrong with abortion, what difference does it make how often abortions occur? Imagine a sexually active person who does not use birth control. If this person begins to be sexually active at 15 and continues through menopause, she could possibly become pregnant three or four times a year (presuming that she has an abortion soon after the beginning of each pregnancy). Each time, she has an abortion, and in the course of her reproductive years this could result in more than 100 abortions, a few every year throughout all the years of her fertility. Consider, on the other hand, someone who begins and successfully uses contraception beginning at 16 through menopause and never has an unwanted pregnancy and so never has an abortion. Are the actions of these two people really morally alike? If there is nothing morally wrong with abortion, then our answer must be "yes." Surely there is a world of moral difference between having 100 abortions and using contraception successfully throughout a lifetime.

Someone might argue that so many abortions are bad for a woman's health, but presumably the moral qualms would not be entirely removed if abortions were as safe as taking aspirin. Further, it is normally pro-life advocates who hold that abortion is dangerous for the psychological and physical health of women, while typical defenders of abortion reject these concerns as unfounded. So the typical defender of abortion cannot appeal to health concerns in order to argue that abortion ought to be rare.

In explaining the difference, one might point out that abortion is more invasive and expensive than contraception. However, such differences do not essentially separate abortion from contraception. One could get a free abortion, and one might have to pay a great deal for a given kind of contraception (e.g., surgical sterilization). Whether a procedure is invasive or not similarly does not properly divide contraception from abortion. Vasectomy and tubal ligation are invasive, but no one argues that they ought to be rare, while certain forms of abortion, like RU-486, are not surgically invasive.

Perhaps other differences account for our intuitions. Bonnie Steinbock notes: "There is no question that abortion is for most women psychologically and emotionally different from contraception. Few women experience abortion as just another way to avoid motherhood" (1992, pp. 66–67). As noted in the discussion of the "Comparative Burdens Objection" (section 7.7), Steinbock is certainly correct about the emotional heartbreak often caused by abortion. The fact that abortion is typically more emotionally difficult than contraception reveals something important. The difference cannot be traced simply to cost or invasiveness. Is not the emotional difficulty of having an abortion typically due to an awareness, however implicit, that whereas contraception prevents a new human life from existing, abortion destroys a new human life? Arguably, the emotional difference is due to a recognition of the moral difference between abortion and contraception, but the moral evil of abortion is precisely what the defender of the moral permissibility of abortion is committed to denying.

8.3.5 Why Personal Opposition?

Finally, many people say that they are personally opposed to abortion but do not want to impose their views on others. I may be personally opposed to being mean to my mother, and yet not want a law that punishes being rude to one's mother. I may choose not to drink alcohol, and yet not be a prohibitionist. To believe some act is morally problematic for me is not to claim that it is morally problematic in itself. Likewise, I may consider abortion to be a choice that I personally would not undertake, but nevertheless could support legal rights to abortion as a matter of public policy or make a judgment that abortion is morally permissible for others.

Critics respond that this view is inherently unstable. Presumably, one's personal opposition to abortion rests on the belief that this procedure is the unjust taking of innocent human life, a grave injustice. By contrast, drinking alcohol is not intrinsically unjust and being mean to one's mother is not gravely unjust. But if one believes that abortion is a grave, intrinsic injustice, then how can one support a regime of law that allow or bring about acts of grave injustice? Don't persons of goodwill have a duty to work to eliminate grave injustice? Are there any other grave injustices that we are excused from working to eliminate? On the other hand, if abortion is morally similar to the removal of a tumor, and therefore is not a grave injustice, then what grounds would one have personally to oppose abortion? The reason for personal opposition (that an innocent human being is killed) should lead to public opposition. If this reason is absent, and abortion does not kill an innocent human person, then the reason for personal opposition to abortion also vanishes.

Princeton's Robert George satirizes the "personally opposed" view as follows:

> I am personally opposed to killing abortionists. However, inasmuch as my personal opposition to this practice is rooted in a sectarian (Catholic) religious belief in the sanctity of human life, I am unwilling to impose it on others who may, as a matter of conscience, take a different view. Of course, I am entirely in favor of policies aimed at removing the root causes of violence against abortionists. Indeed, I would go so far as to support mandatory one-week waiting periods, and even nonjudgmental counseling, for people who are contemplating the choice of killing an abortionist. I believe in policies that reduce the urgent need some people feel to kill abortionists while, at the same time, respecting the rights of conscience of my fellow citizens

who believe that the killing of abortionists is sometimes a tragic necessity—not a good, but a lesser evil. In short, I am moderately pro-choice.

(1994)

George's satire points out the inconsistency of the "personally opposed" position on abortion. If abortion is wrong because it is the unjust killing of an innocent human being, a serious injustice against the vulnerable, then more than personal opposition is called for. In general, good people oppose not just personally and privately but publicly and politically what they take to be serious injustices perpetrated on innocent victims.

However, a pro-choice retort would put the inconsistency on the side of those who are pro-life. If abortion is really unjust killing of an innocent human being, then violence against abortionists in order to stop abortion would seem to be a moral duty. A condemnation of violence against abortionists is itself viewed by some critics as an inconsistency. Hence, it would seem that pro-life people do not really believe that abortion is equivalent to murder (McMahan 2007, p. 7; Stretton 2008, p. 795).

As noted earlier (at the end of section 4.3), killing an innocent person is wrong, and equally wrong, as a violation of the right to life. However, not all such killing is equally wrong, all things considered, in terms of the personal culpability of the agents involved and in terms of the circumstances which render some killings circumstantially worse than others. In terms of risking global instability, killing the President of the United States is worse than killing a regular person. Likewise, it is worse, circumstantially, to kill the father of seven young children than to kill someone without dependents.

A different example may make it clear that believing that abortion is the unjust killing of innocent human beings does not require killing abortionists. Many people believe that the second Iraq war initiated by George W. Bush in 2003 was unjust, and although there is disagreement about the exact body count, there is no doubt that this war has taken the lives of thousands and thousands of innocent people. Were war protesters insincere in their convictions or hypocrites in their actions, since they did not attempt to assassinate President Bush, or any of his generals, or even any of the lower level military personnel who carried out this war? When war protestors do not themselves kill those who wage the war, no one accuses them of not "really" believing the war is unjust or not consistently living out their convictions. Yet, when foes of abortion condemn the killing of abortionists (as do all major pro-life groups), they are accused of not practicing what they preach.

In truth, neither those who protest war nor those who protest abortion are hypocritical in not killing for the sake of their beliefs. Characteristically, those who oppose abortion and those who oppose war agree that violence is not the best solution to problems, including the problems of war and abortion. In addition, many unjust wars are legal according to the juridical statues of a given country, so violence in opposition to war is an act of vigilante justice. Similarly, since abortion is legal in most countries, killing an abortionist is an act of vigilante justice which, like other acts of vigilante justice, is *prima facie* wrong:

> There is no universal moral obligation to prevent all evil. Still less does anyone have the moral authority to prevent evil by any and all means that he or his associates consider necessary. . . . Revolutionary actions, such as killing persons for their crimes (however real the crimes may be), strike at the roots of the order on which the life, liberty, and property of all us depend, and therefore the law cannot tolerate them.
>
> (Canavan 1994)

Violation of the law and violent revolution can be justified in extreme circumstances, but it is tremendously difficult to overcome the presumption against such violence, due to the likelihood of even worse injustices taking place in the breakdown of social order brought about by vigilante justice.

Judith Jarvis Thomson provides another way of affirming the personally opposed but publicly in favor of abortion's moral or legal permissibility. Since there is reasonable disagreement over the issue of the ethical or lawful permissibility of abortion, this reasonable disagreement opens the door for liberty in the decision whether to have an abortion. Thomson's argument has three parts:

> First, restrictive regulation [of abortion] severely constrains women's liberty. Second, severe constraints on liberty may not be imposed in the name of considerations that the constrained are not unreasonable in rejecting. And third, the many women who reject the claim that the fetus has a right to life from the moment of conception are not unreasonable in doing so.
>
> (Thomson 1995, p. 20)

In this manner, Thomson seeks to sidestep the issue of whose views about human life and reproductive choice are correct, leaving room for the endorsement of abortion choice, even by those who believe that abortion, in fact, is unjust killing.

Consider Thomson's argument rewritten. First, restrictive regulation of infanticide severely constrains parental liberty, for such parents are forced to remain at minimum biological parents for as long as the child is alive and many would feel obliged also to be social parents. Second, severe constraints on liberty may not be imposed in the name of considerations that the constrained are not unreasonable in rejecting. For example, a mother of a newborn may not want to raise her baby, and she may not want to choose adoption for a variety of reasons, including her perception that placing a child for adoption makes her a bad mother who abandons her own baby to strangers, the fear of uncertainty for the child's future, and concerns that the child may wish to reestablish a relationship in the future (Swope 1998). And third, many intelligent people (e.g., Tooley, Singer, McMahan, Hassoun, Kriegel, Lindemann and Verkerk, as well as those who practice infanticide) who reject the claim that the infant has a right to life from the moment of birth are not unreasonable in doing so.

Consider the argument rewritten again. First, restrictive regulation of slavery severely constrains a slave owner's liberty. Second, severe constraints on liberty may not be imposed in the name of considerations that the constrained are not unreasonable in rejecting. And third, the many slave owners who reject the claim that the slave has a right to liberty are not unreasonable in doing so.

In all three arguments, much hinges on what is meant by "not unreasonable," or (eliminating the double negative) "reasonable." If "not unreasonable" is defined as whatever views are held by educated, literate, intelligent people, then Thomson's argument justifies permitting abortion, but it equally justifies slavery (at least at certain periods of time) and infanticide. If reasonable is defined in terms of what actually is in conformity with the truth of the matter, and if the truth is not evident, then one has to debate the individual arguments for and against abortion, slavery, and infanticide (Finnis et al. 2001). There were certainly educated, literate, and intelligent people, such as Thomas Jefferson and George Washington, who owned slaves and who would have considered their emancipation a serious imposition on their liberty, in particular on their property rights. Of course, one might say that Thomson's argument is not about the *people* who endorsed slavery being reasonable but the *arguments* in favor of slavery being reasonable. People such as Thomas Jefferson and George Washington were reasonable people in general but not reasonable in rejecting arguments on behalf of liberty for slaves. But to determine whether or not an argument for a claim is reasonable, one must look at the validity and soundness of the arguments for and against that claim. Ultimately, the pro-life and the pro-choice arguments cannot be both reasonable in the sense that arguments on both sides cannot be sound and valid, since the arguments have opposing conclusions. So if Thomson's argument is construed as pertaining to the reasonability of people, it cannot exclude slavery or infanticide. If Thomson's argument is about the reasonability of the arguments, then it must ultimately rest on an analysis of the soundness and validity of these arguments. If these practices are morally permissible in truth, then even if those who consider these practices morally impermissible are reasonable in many respects, they are not reasonable in their moral condemnation of these practices because they are adhering to false conclusions in these matters. If these practices are morally impermissible in truth, then those defending these practices are not reasonable insofar as adhering to false conclusions is unreasonable. So, Thomson's argument either proves too much, that not just abortion but also slavery and infanticide should be permissible or it simply points us back to the arguments for and against such practices.

8.3.6 Prenatal Bonding with "Our Baby"

Those who accept the permissibility of destroying human beings in their embryonic and fetal stages of development typically deny that these human beings are persons in a moral sense. If such human beings are not persons, indeed beings without any moral worth, it is difficult to explain why receptive parents who begin to love their children while they are still in utero are not slipping into a mistaken judgment about the value of these human beings. Many of these parents grieve deeply when struck by miscarriage, but if the early human fetus is of no greater worth than an appendix or a guppy, such people would seem silly and irrational. On the one hand, if such preborn human beings are rightly loved by their parents, then it would seem that these human embryos and fetuses are rightly considered beings of moral worth. On the other hand, if the human fetus lacks moral worth, then such parents are acting irrationally in their joy and care for the "one on the way." Is the early fetus a being that it is appropriate to love for his or her own sake? Or are such human beings without any moral worth?

Elizabeth Harman offers a sophisticated way of accounting for parental bonding by questioning the supposition that each early fetus of similar health and development has the same moral worth. She posits what she calls, "The Ever Conscious View: A being has moral status at a time just in case it is alive at that time and there is a time in its life at which it is conscious" (Harman 2007, p. 220). On this view, if a being is actually conscious in the past, present, or future, then the being has moral status as long as it is alive. To assert that beings have moral status if they are currently conscious is relatively uncontroversial; likewise, to hold that beings have moral status if they have been conscious in the past is likewise fairly uncontroversial (though the moral status of permanently unconscious human beings has been questioned). The new addition to the discussion has to do with future consciousness, what Harman calls elsewhere the Actual Future Principle, "The Actual Future Principle: An early fetus that will become a person has some moral status. An early fetus that will die while it is still an early fetus has no moral status" (Harman 2000, p. 311). If an early fetus has an actual future in which he or she will be conscious, then the human fetus has moral worth. On the other hand, if an early fetus does not have an actual future in which he or she will be conscious, then the human fetus does not have moral worth. In this way, prospective parents who begin to love and value their child as soon as pregnancy begins are acting reasonably, since it is likely that this baby will actually be conscious in the future. On the other hand, having an abortion early in pregnancy destroys a being of no moral worth, since these human beings do not have an actual future in which they will be conscious.

It is important to distinguish this principle from what Harman calls the Mother's Intention Principle which states that "an early fetus has some moral status if and only if the woman pregnant with it is planning to carry it to term" (2000, p. 318). This principle likewise can secure the two intuitions in question: wanted fetuses have moral worth; unwanted fetuses lack moral worth. However, as Harman points out, imagine a women intent on getting an abortion. Her friend talks her out of having an abortion, but then the next day she changes her mind back again. At the abortion clinic door, she decides at the last moment against going into the clinic. The next week she returns and has the abortion. Harman rejects the Mother's Intention Principle because on this view the same fetus would lack moral worth, then have it, lack it again, and then have it again, only to lose it again.

> This is metaphysically absurd; these fluctuations in moral status do not correspond to any fluctuations in anything we might call the fetus's nature. The intentions of the woman who carries a fetus are weak, relational properties of that fetus; they are not among the facts that can determine what kind of thing it is. The Actual Future Principle does not require us to accept any similar metaphysical absurdity. Throughout each fetus's existence as an early fetus, the question whether it has moral status yields a single answer. It does not depend on the day of the week.
>
> (2000, p. 318)

Since this human fetus died, despite all the alternations in the mother's intention, the actual future of this fetus did not include ever being conscious, so the fetus in question was never a being with moral worth.

According to Harman, the actual future of a human fetus is an intrinsic property (unlike the Mother's Intention Principle which is a relational property) determining the nature of the fetus, making the human fetus a particular kind of being. Human fetuses, otherwise alike in terms of health and development, actually come in two kinds, those with an actual future including consciousness and those without an actual future of consciousness. Future consciousness or its lack determines whether the fetus has moral worth now.

One trouble with the Actual Future Principle is that the actual future of any particular fetus is unknown, and since it is unknown the Actual Future Principle cannot serve as a guide to knowing the moral status of the fetus. We cannot know the future of any given human fetus, since some women intent on abortion end up not getting one, and other women intent on keeping their pregnancies lose them. Harman responds to this objection, "we often do know a fetus's overwhelmingly likely future" (2000, p. 319). This adjustment to the Actual Future Principle changes it in substance to the Likely Future Principle. But unlike the Actual Future, the Likely Future of any given being is not fixed but rather a weak, relational property which changes with the circumstances. We can indeed know the Likely Future of any given fetus based at least in part on the mother's intentions, but Harman rightly rejects this as a ground for determining fetal moral status.

A second trouble with the Actual Future Principle is that the "Actual Future" for any given being is a contradiction in terms. Insofar as some characteristic is actual, it is not going to come to be in the future; and insofar as the characteristic is a future characteristic, it cannot be actual now. A being's future is simply not a part of what the being actually is now, its current nature. In other words, a being's future consciousness is not (yet) an inherent property, since inherent properties are actual properties and what is future is not yet actual.

A third trouble with the Actual Future Principle is that even if we could know the future of any given fetus, and even if a being's "Actual Future" were not a contradiction in terms, this future insofar as it is future cannot determine the nature of the being in question now. Indeed, it is the nature of the being in question that determines its future possibilities rather than the future possibilities determining the nature of the being in question now (Tollefsen 2008, pp. 46–47).

A fourth challenge rests on distinguishing extrinsic, intrinsic, and essential properties. As Tollefsen notes:

> Being loved by Smith is an extrinsic property, but having blue eyes seems to be an intrinsic property of me, but not an essential property; that property could be lost without my ceasing to be me. Similarly, my being conscious right now is an intrinsic property, but it is not an essential property, as Harman would also surely allow: I do not cease to be—there is no essential change—if I cease to be conscious (through, for example, a temporary coma). The question about our nature should be framed first, then, not in terms of intrinsic properties, but in terms of essential properties—those properties the possession of which is necessary for me to remain a being of the same essential sort that I am now, and hence, those properties possession of which is necessary for me to remain me. It must be *these* properties that we focus on if we are concerned with the question of moral status and want to honor Harman's claim that moral status must be determined by a thing's *nature*.
>
> (2008, p. 46)

Intrinsic properties—such as eye color or consciousness—cannot define our nature, since our nature—our essential properties—determines what kind of intrinsic properties we can have, rather than our intrinsic properties determining what kind of nature we have.

Finally, Harman's view does not in fact fully make sense of parents' prenatal bonding. The Actual Future Principle can make sense of the love that many couples experience for their offspring prior to birth, so long as these children live to be conscious. The Actual Future Principle still cannot account for the grief that many couples have at miscarriage. A human fetus who dies in utero, whether from abortion or spontaneous miscarriage, has no Actual Future Consciousness and so, on Harman's view, had no moral worth. But many parents grieve over the loss of a pregnancy, not merely as contradiction to their own plans, and not merely as they would have had conception not taken place. Rather, they grieve the loss of someone who mattered for himself or herself. In other words, they grieve the loss of someone who had moral status. Harman's account still views such grieving parents as silly and irrational for making a fuss over nothing morally significant.

8.3.7 *Morally Permissible vs. Morally Objectionable*

Perhaps we could draw a distinction between being *morally permissible* and *morally objectionable* in order to respond to many of the hard cases for defenders of abortion. According to this view, abortion is ethically permissible, but nevertheless still morally objectionable. Pro-choice advocates might disagree as to what counts as objectionable, with some holding that all abortions are objectionable, but others holding that just some, like for sex selection or trivial reasons, are objectionable. For example, someone adopting Thomson's argument for abortion (rather than a denier of fetal personhood) could respond that sex selection abortion is similar to unplugging yourself from the violinist simply because you found out that it was a female violinist rather than a male violinist. You have no obligation to remain plugged into the violinist but to unplug yourself for the reason that it is a female rather than a male violinist is morally objectionable. A pro-choice advocate could generalize this principle to all abortions. According to this view, it is morally permissible to have an abortion, and so abortions should be legal; but it is also morally objectionable to have an abortion, so abortion should be rare.

In ethical terms, I'm not sure that this distinction is a real one. There is a distinction between morally permissible and morally heroic action, between the obligatory and the supererogatory acts. But if the analysis given earlier is correct (sections 7.4–7.8) then it is not accurate to think about abortion in terms of these categories. There is also a distinction between actions that are seriously wrong (assault, violations of the right to life) and actions that are wrong but not seriously wrong (rudeness, inconsiderateness). If an action is morally objectionable, that is, if a moral objection is a sound objection, then the action is either seriously morally wrong or morally wrong but not seriously morally wrong. If the moral objection is not a sound one, then the action is not morally wrong in either sense. Further, if abortion is wrong as violation of the right to live, then it falls into the category of actions that are seriously wrong rather than into the category of actions that are not seriously wrong. If abortion is not morally wrong, then there can be no sound moral objection to it, so the category of morally objectionable does not apply to it.

8.3.8 Intermediate Moral Worth of the Human Fetus

Now the defender of abortion can respond to all these cases with one rejoinder. The murder of pregnant women, a condemnation of sex selection abortion, the moral impermissibility of abortion for insignificant reasons, personal opposition, the desire to see the practice of abortion become rare, and parental love for their prenatal children do not presuppose the personhood of the fetus, but rather that the human fetus has some value. So these cases provide a difficulty for the view that the human fetus has no moral worth whatsoever, but provide no difficulty for the view that the human in utero has some value, albeit not a value equal to a full human person. One could argue for example that a puppy dog has some moral worth and so should not be destroyed simply because of its sex or for frivolous reasons, and so forth. Nothing in this response presupposes that a puppy has equal moral worth to a human person. Likewise, a human fetus, if it has some worth, would merit the kind of consideration due to the puppy, not the absolute respect due a person but more respect than is due a being with no moral worth, such as a cockroach or a blade of grass.

The strength of this response depends on how the moral worth of the human fetus is established. For some, the biological humanity of the fetus alone would establish some worth or perhaps the potentiality of the human fetus to develop into an adult human being. Others could point to sentience as the characteristic granting moral worth. Still others could argue that increasing physiological or psychological development is linked to increasing moral worth (the developmental, pluralistic view). In effect, this position returns us to the many arguments about personhood presented in previous chapters of this book, with two important differences: first, "moral worth" would be substituted for "personhood", and second, the pro-choice advocate would be in the position of defending the moral worth of the human fetus against various objections. In other words, the defender of abortion will have to simultaneously attack the personhood of the human fetus and defend the moral worth of the human fetus.

I am skeptical that the intermediate "moral worth" of the human fetus can be successfully defended from a typical pro-choice perspective. "On any fair comparison of morally relevant characteristics, like rationality, self-consciousness, awareness, autonomy, pleasure and pain, and so on," writes Peter Singer, "the calf, the pig and the much derided chicken come out well ahead of the fetus at any stage of pregnancy" (1993, p. 151). Or, as Warren puts the point, "in the relevant respects, a fetus, *even a fully developed one*, is considerably less person-like than the average mammal, indeed the average fish" (1973, pp. 264–265, emphasis added). So, if their case for undermining personhood succeeds, the "moral worth" of the fetus does not render abortion morally problematic. Since the human fetus is, according to Warren, less a person than the average fish, whatever would justify a fishing trip would also justify a visit to an abortion clinic, even in the third trimester of pregnancy.

The critiques of conceptions of personhood offered in previous chapters can usually also be applied to appeal to the same standards to justify lesser degrees of moral worth. Consider, for example, Bonnie Steinbock's argument against frivolous uses of the human fetus:

> On the interest view, preconscious fetuses are not human subjects whose consent must be secured in order to use them in experiments. Restrictions on such research cannot stem from concern for fetal welfare. However, nonsentient fetuses can be respected as a symbol of human life, and restrictions may legitimately be placed on fetal research and the use of fetal tissue, so long as this respect does not interfere with the real interests of actual people.
>
> (1992, p. 7)

In this passage, what is given on the one hand is taken away with the other, for since the real interests of actual people always trump the symbolic value of human life, it is hard to conceive of a realistic example of someone wanting to experiment on a dead or even a living human fetus that would not be validated by this standard. A crash test dummy and a painting of a human being also symbolize human life (more recognizably than does the immature fetus or embryo), but surely respect for neither needs to interrupt virtually any of our plans or experiments.

Another possible response to hard cases for advocates of abortion is to liken abortion to inflicting pain upon or euthanizing a dog or cat. It is not that the dog or cat is the moral equal to a human person, but nevertheless inflicting pain on an animal is a regretful situation that should be avoided when possible since the dog or cat has some moral status in virtue of being a sentient being. For the same reason, it is wrong to intentionally cause a dog or cat to suffer, not because they are persons but because suffering is bad for any sentient being, human or non-human.

This response does not really explain why abortion for frivolous reasons or sex selection should be considered morally tragic, regrettable, or problematic. According to most defenders of abortion, sentience occurs very late in pregnancy and so, in their view, 99% of abortions do not in fact harm a sentient being. So, while there is reason to be concerned with the dog and the cat (both of which are actually sentient beings) only a late-term abortion would be cause for concern. Even in late-term abortion, the fetus could be anesthetized before being killed which would eliminate the concern for causing pain. Thus, late-term abortion would be problematic not in itself, but only as currently practiced because abortion inflicts pain on the human fetus.

Another difficulty with likening the worth of the human fetus to a dog or a cat is that the intermediate status assigned dogs and cats does not seem adequate to secure protection of their interests in the first place. I mean not simply that animals are often treated in disrespectful ways, though that is true. The difficulty is that the allegedly intermediate status of non-human animals fails to provide a sound basis for ethical critiques of their misuse. As Gary Francione notes:

> We tried, through slavery welfare laws, to have a three-tiered system: things, or inanimate property; persons, who were free, and in the middle, depending on your choice of locution, "quasi-persons" or "things plus"—the slaves. That system could not work. We eventually recognized that if slaves were going to have morally significant interests, they could not be slaves any more, for the moral universe is limited to only two kinds of beings: persons and things. "Quasi-persons" or "things plus" will necessarily risk being treated as things because the principle of equal consideration cannot apply to them. Nor can we use animal welfare laws to render animals "quasi-persons" or "things plus." They are either persons, beings to whom the principle of equal consideration applies and who possess morally significant interests in not suffering, or things, beings to whom the principle of equal consideration does not apply and whose interests may be ignored if it benefits us. There is no third choice.
>
> (2004, p. 131)

If the third choice, neither persons nor things but quasi-persons, is not open for animals, neither is it open for immature human beings in or out of the uterus.

But why not a middle ground in which non-human animals and fetuses do not have a right to life, but nevertheless do have interests which should be taken into account? A middle view could be carved out in which the interests of the pig and the fetus do not count equally but do count in part against the interests of the adult human.

In this kind of view, we have to consider what interest it is that the pig and the fetus have. Many pro-choice advocates, such as Singer and Warren, consider the interests of the fetus to be less than a pig or a fish, so, on this view, fetal interests will hardly be weighty enough to do the work required to render problematic any abortion.

On the other hand, if somehow the intermediate moral worth of the human fetus is truly established, this may prove too much. If the moral worth of the human fetus is going to do the required work of rendering problematic, say sex selection abortion, consistently applied this account of moral status may in fact lead to a condemnation of more abortions than the typical pro-choice advocate would wish. The interest of the fetus in living (objectively considered, not subjectively considered) are as weighty as any interest can be, for in losing life what is also lost is all other interests that currently exist or will exist in the future. So, if these interests count, unless they are weighted in such a way that they barely count at all or do not count, it is hard to see how these interests could be outweighed by anything short of the life of the adult human. Indeed, if the moral worth of the human fetus is truly robust, this worth may not differ in a significant way from considering the human fetus a person.

An example of instability of such compromises is Christopher Nobbs's article, "Probability Potentiality," which attempts to secure some value for human non-persons, such as infants (2007). Nobbs holds that actual persons must be self-aware, but also that those who are potential persons in his view—such as human babies—have some value because they are highly likely to achieve personhood. A lottery ticket with a fifty–fifty chance of being worth a million dollars is extremely valuable (as calculated by rational decision theory, 50% × $1,000,000 = $500,000). However, this lottery ticket is not as valuable as one million dollars itself. So too the human infant is not equal to a person and yet is of such high value that parents may not neglect or kill the child because of the probability that the infant will become a person. With this application of a kind of rational decision theory to the question of when human life becomes valuable, Nobbs attempts to maintain the self-awareness view of personhood and yet not sanction the moral permissibility of infant neglect.

Several difficulties face this proposal. Obviously, the probability of an infant reaching personhood must be conceived of independently of detrimental human intervention. Otherwise, parents could neglect or kill the infant at will, since the probability of such an infant reaching personhood with the harmful human intervention would be quite low, if not zero. If harmful human choices are excluded from the probability, then it is difficult to see why the human fetus—from quite early in pregnancy—would be much different than the human newborn. After a pregnancy is well established, miscarriage—like stillbirth or SIDS—is relatively rare, so the human fetus would seem to have a high likelihood of reaching personhood and so would have a high value. This would seem to exclude abortion save for the most serious of reasons, if not, then one would have to endorse infanticide for birth control and convenience as takes place in most abortions. In other words, if potential value is going to do the work needed to exclude infant neglect or infanticide, this value will also interfere with many abortions—presumably a view that Nobbs does not want to embrace given his endorsement of something like Singer's view of personhood, a view typically driven by the desire to justify abortion.

Another difficulty is that in any calculus of probability and value both terms are relevant. In other words, in terms of shifting the outcome, if a value is high enough, even a low probability yields high probability value. So in adjudicating among various options, not simply the probability but also the value involved is relevant. Considering negative outcomes, it would be irrational for me to wager even with good odds, if losing the wager would result in, say, thermonuclear destruction of the entire earth. Put positively, if the value of personhood is high enough, even a low probability of achieving personhood yields great value which would again seems to lead to a condemnation of not just infanticide but also abortion. If we affirm the incomparable value of every actual human person, then this inestimable value shifts the probability calculus decidedly against negative interventions against "potential" persons even in the face of low probability.

Considered from another perspective, Nobbs's view of probability potentiality is unlikely to be firm ground to demonstrate the problematic nature of infanticide or infant neglect to many pro-choice advocates. Commenting on her own example of a space explorer whose body contains virtually millions of potential persons, Mary Anne Warren, as noted in chapter three, has remarked that the rights of an actual person always outweigh the rights of however many potential persons (1973, pp. 265–266). If so, then it is difficult to see what practical difference it would make if infants (or other human beings) have greater value the more likely it is that they are to achieve personhood. It would still be permissible for a couple to take a vacation, leaving their newborn at home to die from neglect, since the rights and desires of actual persons could in principle never be outweighed by the rights and desires of non-persons however close to achieving personhood.

Although there are "hard cases" for both those who support and those who reject abortion, speaking of hard cases of abortion is in a sense a misnomer. Abortion is not chosen (at least normally) as a positive good, like food or recreation. In the vast majority of cases, abortion is regretfully carried out as a last resort that would not have been chosen in other circumstances. I believe that this is due to the implicit recognition even by those who undergo and perform abortions that abortion ends the life of innocent human beings, a morally problematic act. What we have discussed in this chapter, then, are extremely difficult cases of abortion. Is there any possible way of solving such cases to the satisfaction of virtually everyone, both those that describe themselves as pro-life and those that describe themselves as pro-choice? The next chapter discusses on such possibility.

9   Could Artificial Wombs End the Abortion Debate?

Although artificial wombs may seem fanciful when first considered, it is difficult to know what scientists will invent. If artificial wombs were made available, relatively affordable and the procedure was no more intrusive than present day abortion, would abortion defenders be satisfied with abortion extraction (removing the living human fetus for implantation in an artificial womb) or would they insist on the right to abortion termination (ending human fetal life)? Would the use of an artificial womb in lieu of abortion be morally permissible for ardent critics of abortion? Or, would religious teaching, if only implicitly, exclude this practice? Depending on how these questions are answered, it could be the case that most ardent critics of abortion and most ardent defenders of abortion could both be satisfied, and the abortion debate among intellectuals at least as we know it now would change profoundly if not altogether be ended. Needless to say, my remarks here are necessarily "exploratory" insofar as they try to reason about non-existent technology. It would be extremely difficult, if not impossible, beforehand to explore in depth the political, social, and economic ramifications of an artificial uterus, and yet an admittedly incomplete consideration of the ethical dimensions of this possibility may better prepare us, if this possibility ever becomes a reality.

9.1   Artificial Wombs and Ardent Defenders of Abortion

Ardent defenders of abortion believe that abortion is morally permissible in all circumstances throughout all nine months of pregnancy. In legal and sometime also moral terms, ardent defenders of abortion assert an absolute right to abortion, even as ardent critics of abortion defend an exceptionless norm against intentionally killing the human fetus. But what exactly is meant by the "right to abortion"?

One should distinguish two aspects of abortion that are currently but not necessarily linked—extraction and termination. Abortion rights might be understood as the right not to be pregnant, the right not to have the human fetus in the womb, the right of extraction. On the other hand, abortion rights might be defined as the right to end the life of the human fetus in utero, the right to terminate not just the pregnancy but also the fetus. These two understandings of abortion, though distinct, are at least for the present linked, since one cannot currently accomplish evacuation of the human fetus from the uterus at an early stage of pregnancy without also terminating the life of the human fetus. Accordingly, one could advocate the right of evacuation or extraction, that is, the right to have the fetus removed from the woman's body, and yet not advocate a right of termination, that is the right to have the fetus killed within the woman's body. The question then can be asked: When someone defends the right to an abortion, does this include only evacuation or also termination?

From my reading, most defenders of abortion in fact only advocate a right to evacuation and not a right to termination. For example, in 1977 ACOG wrote:

> The College affirms that the resolution of such conflict (between woman and fetus) by inducing abortion in no way implies that the physician has an adversary relationship towards the fetus and therefore, the physician does not view the destruction of the fetus as the primary purpose of abortion. The College consequently recognizes a continuing obligation on the part of the physician towards the survival of a possibly viable fetus where this can be discharged without additional hazard to the health of the mother.
>
> (cited by Nathanson 1979, pp. 179–180)

If methods of non-lethal evacuation were available and safe for maternal health, then this statement would require that doctors use these means. Artificial wombs as envisioned are precisely means that would enable the survival of a viable fetus without additional hazard to the health of the mother. If all physicians abided by this statement, this alone would dramatically change the abortion debate, for if the medical community refused to perform terminal abortions and would only perform evacuation abortions, then the abortion debate as we know it today would be over.

Among philosophers defending abortion, many of the most prominent such as Mary Ann Warren, Judith Jarvis Thomson, and David Boonin understand the right to abortion as a *right of evacuation* and *not a right of termination*. In Thomson's words:

> While I am arguing for the permissibility of abortion in some cases, I am not arguing for the right to secure the death of the preborn child. It is easy to confuse these two things in that up to a certain point in the life of the foetus it is not able to survive outside the mother's body; hence removing it from her body guarantees death. But they are importantly different.
>
> (Thomson 1971, p. 66)

Along the same lines, Mary Anne Warren writes:

> If and when a late-term abortion could be safely performed without killing the fetus, she would have no absolute right to insist on its death (e.g., if others wish to adopt it or pay for its care), for the same reason that she does not have a right to insist that a viable infant be killed.
>
> (1973, p. 267)

Warren believes that the rights of the fetus to be in the womb do not trump the woman's right of freedom, which is violated by the pregnancy. However, if the fetus were removed and placed in an artificial womb, the rights of the woman would no longer be violated. Likewise in his book *A Defense of Abortion*, David Boonin argues against abortion as termination:

> The claim that the woman has such a right [to terminating fetal life] would entail that if the baby survived an attempted abortion, or was born prematurely, before the woman had an opportunity to have the abortion performed, then she would still have the right to have it killed. And this is plainly unacceptable. It may well be true that many women who seek abortions do so because they want the fetus that they are carrying to be killed. And such women will, to that extent, be dissatisfied with a position on which it is morally permissible for them to have their viable fetuses extracted but not killed. But in the absence of an independent reason to think that they are entitled to have the fetus die when it is already viable, this seems to count more as a criticism of their desires than as an objection to the good Samaritan argument.
>
> (2003, p. 257)

So, these prominent defenders of abortion defend only a right of evacuation not a right of termination. Safe, practical artificial wombs should therefore end the abortion debate for them. An added advantage, from their perspective, would be that the right to evacuation abortion would be relatively, if not absolutely, uncontested unlike the present, heavily contested abortions, heavily contested because they include termination of the life of the human fetus.

The statement from the American College of Obstetricians and Gynecologists implicitly raises an important objection namely that partial ectogenesis could be more dangerous for the woman and therefore abortion as termination would be preferable. In the words of David N. James:

> A foetal transplant would be an elaborate surgical procedure aimed at the delicate removal of the foetus from the mother's placenta and

its transfer and attachment to the external artificial womb. Unlike an early abortion, foetal transplantation would thus require general anesthesia as well as a surgical incision through the abdominal wall and uterus, with all the risks of medical complications which accompany these more invasive procedures.

(1987, p. 87)

James also notes that intensive care for such children could be massively expensive and lead to many new orphanages, foster care homes, and related services.

These possible difficulties may or may not be realized. If these difficulties were to take place, they would be technological, economic, or social difficulties and not per se moral difficulties. The foreseen social cost of extraction rather than termination may or may not take place. *Ex hypothesis*, partial ectogenesis, as imagined in the future, would not be dangerous for women. Many procedures that were dangerous and invasive 40 years ago now are safe and non-invasive. Many surgeries formerly requiring days in the hospital have become outpatient surgeries. The choice between termination and extraction would not be the choice between no danger and danger, but between two choices, both risking dangers. As medical care advances, it is highly likely that the differences in danger among the various procedures will be negligible, as well as the cost for such treatments less expensive—as is seen, for example, in the cheap, fast, and powerful computers of today when compared with the expensive, slow, and relatively powerless computers of the 1970s. Of course, a cataclysmic disaster could return humanity to the Stone Age, but if the past is any indication of the future, the projected course of technological development strongly suggests that the technological and economic problems that James foresees could be overcome.

Of course, not all doctors, philosophers, or activists defending abortion understand abortion rights in terms of evacuation rather than termination. For some, "abortion rights" includes the right to secure the death of the human fetus. However, even among advocates of infanticide, there is a recognition that insisting on fetal death in the context of artificial wombs might be going too far. As Peter Singer and Deane Wells wrote:

> Freedom to choose what is to happen to one's body is one thing; freedom to insist on the death of a being that is capable of living outside of one's body is another. . . . [Even if there is no fetal right to life] it is difficult to see why a healthy foetus should die if there is someone who wishes to adopt it and will give it the opportunity of a worthwhile life. We do not allow a mother to kill her newborn baby because she does not wish either to keep it or to hand it over for adoption. Unless we were to change our mind about this, it is difficult to see why we should give this right to a woman in respect

of a foetus she is carrying, if her desire to be rid of the foetus can be fully satisfied without threatening the life of the foetus.

(1984, pp. 135–136)

If ardent advocates of abortion and even infanticide such as Peter Singer can embrace the use of advanced incubators in lieu of abortion, then it is likely that there will be few advocates of abortion who will disagree. At least if advocates of abortion such as these are consistent, and really meant what they have said about not desiring the death of the human fetus, for at least these defenders of abortion, artificial wombs would end the abortion debate. An interesting and related question concerns not intellectual defenses of abortion, such as those given by Singer, Boonin, Thomson, Warren, and others, but the political and social advocates of abortion. Here, the possibility of ending the debate is, I'm afraid, much less likely as is evident in some popular reflections on the topic such as Zimmerman's "The Fetal Position" (2003).

9.2 Artificial Wombs and Ardent Critics of Abortion

Ardent critics of abortion hold that intentionally killing a human fetus, as a means or as an end, is always morally wrong. Would the use of artificial wombs be permissible in lieu of abortion for consistent critics of abortion? Several important arguments against artificial wombs have been raised. (For a slightly fuller version of these objections, with citations to those who hold these positions, see Kaczor 2005.) However, I believe that each objection fails and that the use of artificial wombs in lieu of abortion is morally permissible.

By complete ectogenesis, I mean the generation and development of a human being outside the womb from the beginning of embryonic existence until the equivalent of 40 weeks gestation. By partial ectogenesis, I mean the development of a human being during the typical gestational period outside the maternal womb for part but not during the entire gestational period. An artificial womb might be used for complete or partial ectogenesis. It could be used to generate and sustain development of an embryo or fetus during the entire period of gestation or it might be used to sustain development after partial development within the maternal womb. Embryo transfer (ET) moves the human embryo, having never been planted in a womb, to another location, such as an artificial womb or maternal womb. Fetal transfer (FT) moves the fetus from a maternal womb to another maternal womb or to an artificial womb. So, let us now consider some of the likely objections to artificial wombs.

9.2.1 The Artificiality Objection

One possible objection against artificial wombs arises precisely because these wombs are artificial. As artificial, fabricated products, ectogenesis of any kind would be against nature. Since human beings should act in accordance with nature, artificial wombs are impermissible.

However, the "artificiality" of such wombs is not sufficient grounds for rejecting their use. Advanced Neonatal Intensive Care Units are highly "artificial," making use of cutting edge technology of all kinds, but NICUs are not ethically impermissible. Indeed, the artificial wombs envisioned by researchers are nothing more than extremely advanced versions of incubators routinely used today.

Indeed, one can fairly easily imagine artificial wombs that would be acceptable to everyone. Imagine a woman greatly desiring to have children who discovers she has uterine cancer and must have her uterus removed in order to save her life. Portions of a woman's healthy uterine tissue could be used to fashion an artificial uterus for her that could be transplanted back into her own body restoring her fertility. If successful, her womb would be "artificial," fashioned by human hands outside the human body using advanced technology, and yet presumably no more morally problematic than an artificial heart.

9.2.2 The IVF Objection

This objection against artificial wombs arises from opposition to *in vitro* fertilization. If critics oppose IVF, then they should also oppose ectogenesis, since ectogenesis presupposes the use of cloning, parthenogenesis, or IVF in creating an embryo. If ectogenesis is wrong, and the use of artificial wombs in lieu of abortion is a form of ectogenesis, our question has been answered.

However, this objection fails to distinguish between partial ectogenesis and complete ectogenesis. A woman tempted to seek abortion *already has a human fetus within her*. Complete ectogenesis is already excluded. Partial ectogenesis is the continued development of an already generated human being in an artificial womb after transfer from a maternal womb. By definition, partial ectogenesis does not involve generation and development *entirely outside* the womb. So although people who oppose IVF, twin fission, cloning or parthenogenesis, to be consistent should also oppose complete ectogenesis, it does not necessarily follow that they would oppose partial ectogenesis.

9.2.3 The Deprivation of Maternal Shelter Objection

The *deprivation of maternal shelter* objection is more difficult. Someone might hold that the human fetus is wronged in being deprived of maternal shelter. Partial ectogenesis necessarily involves the deprivation of maternal shelter and gestation, and so the use of artificial wombs would seem to be objectionable.

It is possible, however, that deprivation of maternal shelter and gestation is *prima facie* wrong, but nevertheless may be justified in certain circumstances. Consider the case of a woman with a premature but viable baby who begins to die, or actually dies. Surgeons on hand rush to remove the premature baby, depriving him or her of maternal gestation, but of course this removal is not in itself morally objectionable. One can imagine other situations where a preborn child must be removed from the uterus or else he or she will die, such as a mother with an incompetent uterus or a situation in which the mother has been poisoned, and the poison will kill the child unless it is immediately removed from the womb. In these cases, removing the child from the maternal womb does no offense against the dignity of the child. Maternal gestation and shelter are important to the human being in utero to the extent that they aid and support the well-being of the human fetus. In cases where it endangers the life of a human being to remain in utero, depriving a human fetus of maternal gestation is not morally objectionable, but may be morally praiseworthy.

Of course, all the cases appealed to in the previous paragraph involve medical pathology threatening fetal life rather than a free choice of the will. If natural causes endanger the life of the human fetus, then removal is permissible and depravation of maternal gestation does not offend the dignity of the human being in utero. On the other hand, if the life of the human fetus is threatened by the choice of abortion, deprivation of maternal gestation is blameworthy. Depriving the human being in utero of care and shelter may be permissible in the first case of natural causes, but not permissible in the second case where the danger to the child is voluntarily caused and could be voluntarily removed.

Does the voluntary or involuntary nature of the danger mark a morally decisive difference between the two cases? Whether the danger is voluntarily or non-voluntarily caused makes no difference from the perspective of the preborn who are threatened with death. Death is just as final if from a voluntary cause as from a non-voluntary cause. Indeed many "natural" causes of danger to the human fetus are themselves in origin voluntarily caused. For example, one can imagine cases in which the pregnant woman is dying because she was in a car accident that she caused by her irresponsible driving, or perhaps the woman is dying from lung cancer because she smoked cigarettes. The details of the causal chain that ends with a human fetus being in danger of death unless removed from the womb do not, therefore, appear to be morally decisive in determining the permissibility of the use of highly advanced incubators.

Another important distinction between the two cases, partial ectogenesis instead of abortion on the one hand and on the other hand fetal removal on account of a maternal pathology threatening fetal well-being, is that in the first case the removal is motivated by the (perceived) well-being of the mother, but in the second the removal is motivated by the well-being of the child. Perhaps this difference could account for the impermissibility of the first act but the clear permissibility of the second.

However, there are other cases, not normally viewed as problematic, in which the removal of the child takes place for the well-being of the woman. In the case of a gravid cancerous uterus, the removal of uterus and child takes place to preserve the mother's, not the child's well-being. According to widely accepted understandings of double-effect reasoning, the removal of the gravid cancerous uterus is morally permissible even if the premature child would die. If fetal viability has already been achieved, the removal is even easier to justify. For a variety of reasons, some of which are legitimate and will be discussed below, many women choose to induce labor so as to deliver their babies before their due date. It seems that there is tacit agreement that such practices are morally unproblematic so long as the safety of the mother and child is not endangered. Some women are induced because they have extremely rapid labors; others due to their discomfort near the end of pregnancy; still others for reasons entirely unrelated to physical well-being such as the preference for a certain date of birth for their child. None of these practices are impermissible. If ectogenesis functions as envisioned, then induction of labor or surgical removal of the human fetus at any stage of pregnancy could become no less dangerous than induction of pregnancy is now with contemporary technology a few days before the due date. In such circumstances, whatever would justify delivering a child a few days earlier, which is virtually anything, would also justify ectogenesis.

This arguably proves too much, for even if partial ectogenesis might be permissible in lieu of abortion, it seems *prima facie* morally problematic to choose partial ectogenesis for trivial reasons. One might then carve out a "middle position" such that partial ectogenesis ought *not* to be used for utterly trivial reasons, and yet *may* be chosen in circumstances in which a person might otherwise be tempted to choose abortion. It would be difficult, if not impossible to detail all the circumstances. However, one might liken the use of partial ectogenesis to adoption generally. It would be wrong to place a child in another family in an adoption simply because the child's birthday fell on the "wrong" day or because one did not want to suffer trivial inconvenience. On the other hand, adoption in other circumstances, such as when a judgment is made that the child's best interests would be served by adoption, is fully permissible. Generally, the bond between mother and child should not be broken, but given due circumstances both adoption as we now know it and partial ectogenesis as it has been imagined here, are permissible despite undermining the natural mother–child bond.

9.2.4 *The Birth Within Marriage Objection*

The right of a child to be born within marriage is another objection that could be raised to the use of highly advanced incubators in the context of possible abortion. In the words of *Donum vitae*:

Techniques of fertilization *in vitro* can open the way to other forms of biological and genetic manipulation of human embryos, such as attempts or plans for fertilization between human and animal gametes and the gestation of human embryos in the uterus of animals, or the hypothesis or project of constructing artificial uteruses for the human embryo. These procedures are contrary to the human dignity proper to the embryo, and at the same time they are contrary to the right of every person to be conceived and to be born within marriage and from marriage.

(CDF 1987, section I.6)

This passage is particularly noteworthy in that it explicitly mentions the possibility of constructing artificial uteruses and seems to condemn ectogenesis.

Indeed, this passage of *Donum vitae* clearly indicates the moral impermissibility of complete ectogenesis, but it does not necessarily exclude partial ectogenesis. Whenever the human fetus leaves his or her mother's womb, whether by surgical intervention or naturally, whether full term or earlier, a human being can rightly be said to be born. Unlike complete ectogenesis condemned by this passage, partial ectogenesis takes place after human birth, albeit a preterm, voluntarily initiated human birth. Hence, partial ectogenesis is simply not within the scope of this passage from *Donum vitae*, which discusses the right to be born within marriage.

9.2.5 The Integrative Parenthood Objection

Donum vitae clarifies the meaning of the right to be born within marriage in the following passage in ways that would seem to also exclude partial ectogenesis. Call this the *integrative parenthood* objection to partial ectogenesis.

The child has the right to be conceived, *carried in the womb*, brought into the world and brought up within marriage: it is through the secure and recognized relationship to his own parents that the child can discover his own identity and achieve his own proper human development.

(CDF 1987, section II.1)

Artificial insemination using egg or sperm from someone outside the marriage is also impermissible for the same reason:

Heterologous artificial fertilization violates the rights of the child; it deprives him of his filial relationship with his parental origins and can hinder the maturing of his personal identity. Furthermore, it offends the common vocation of the spouses who are called to fatherhood and motherhood: it objectively deprives conjugal fruitfulness of its unity and integrity; it brings about and manifests a rupture between genetic parenthood, gestational parenthood, and responsibility for upbringing.

(CDF 1987, section II.2)

At first glance, these passages seem clearly to exclude partial ectogenesis as undermining *gestational parenthood*, which is important in securing the well-being of the child. Integrative parenthood involves not separating genetic parenthood, gestational parenthood, and what might be called social parenthood, namely the responsibility for raising and rearing the child. A child has a right to *integrative parenthood*, and even partial ectogenesis violates this right by depriving the human fetus of gestational parenthood.

However, this interpretation of the importance of integrative parenthood cannot be maintained. If a right to be conceived, gestated, and raised within marriage were understood to mean that every child *once conceived* must be brought up within marriage, it would follow that all women who find themselves pregnant outside of marriage (even by incestuous rape) must marry the father. In many cases of extramarital pregnancy, a marriage of father and mother constitutes the best response to the situation. However, marriage following pregnancy is not always advisable, let alone a moral duty. Indeed in at least some cases of extra-marital pregnancy, marriage is not only gravely imprudent but indeed is not permissible or even possible, such as when a pregnancy occurs as the result of incest or when a prior valid marriage exists for one or both of the parties in question or when a pregnancy arises involving a party of very young age. In addition, if the right to integrative parenthood were interpreted as the right of every existing child to be nurtured in his or her mother's womb until full-term birth and then raised in a marriage, then every birth mother placing a child for adoption and every couple accepting an adopted child would be acting impermissibly. Of course, given due circumstances, birth parents and adoptive parents do nothing wrong in their acts of giving and receiving the child. Indeed, birth mothers act generously and bravely in placing their child in another family through adoption. When adoption is in the child's best interest, birth mothers perform a loving and heroic act and those who adopt children likewise perform a generous act. *Donum vitae* itself notes that adoption is an important service to life:

Physical sterility in fact can be for spouses the occasion for other important services to the life of the human person, for example, adoption, various forms of educational work, and assistance to other families and to poor or handicapped children.

(CDF 1987, section II.8)

A child's right to integrative parenthood is misinterpreted if this right would lead to a condemnation of adoption.

Donum vitae's right to integrative parenthood should be understood as positing that one should not *cause a human being to come into existence* unless one can properly care for the child. A child's right to integrative parenthood means that parents should not set out to conceive a child unless there is a marriage of the child's mother and father, conception by mother and father in the act of marriage, the intention to nurture within the maternal womb, and then to raise the child within marriage. However, *once conception of a new human being has taken place*, inside of marriage or outside, it is in certain circumstances permissible, and even praiseworthy, to choose adoption, if this option is judged by sound prudential judgment to be in the best interest of the individual child. Although it would be wrong to conceive a child simply in order to place him or her for adoption, virtually everyone's support of adoption makes it clear that, it is not wrong to choose adoption following the conception of a child. Whether this adoption takes place at a few weeks after birth, at 40 weeks of full gestation, at 25 weeks following conception on account of premature birth, or at seven weeks following conception does not, in itself, seem morally relevant so long as the well-being of the child is not endangered. The right to integrative parenthood does not exclude adoption and would seem also not to exclude partial ectogenesis.

9.2.6 The Surrogate Motherhood Objection

The surrogate motherhood objection would describe ectogenesis as a form of surrogate motherhood. Some people who oppose abortion also oppose surrogate motherhood. For example, *Donum vitae* clearly teach that surrogate motherhood is ethically impermissible.

> Surrogate motherhood represents an objective failure to meet the obligations of maternal love, of conjugal fidelity, and of responsible motherhood; it offends the dignity and the right of the child to be conceived, carried in the womb, brought into the world and brought up by his own parents; it sets up, to the detriment of families, a division between the physical, psychological and moral elements which constitute those families.
>
> (CDF 1987, section II.3)

If surrogate motherhood is wrong, and if ectogenesis is a form of surrogate motherhood, indeed an artificial surrogate motherhood, then ectogenesis would also be wrong. This might be called the *surrogate motherhood objection* to the use of highly advanced incubators in lieu of abortion.

In response, it should be noted that in neither of the definitions given in *Donum vitae* (II.3) would partial ectogenesis count as a form of surrogate motherhood, since both definitions speak of transfer of an embryo but in partial ectogenesis no embryo but rather a fetus is transferred. In addition, both definitions of surrogate motherhood involve promises made by the surrogate mother to give up the baby once it is born to whoever commissioned or made the agreement for pregnancy. Obviously, an artificial womb cannot pledge or agree to anything, nor must partial ectogenesis involve giving the baby to those who initiated creation of the baby. Indeed, in cases where partial ectogenesis is chosen instead of abortion, the woman who otherwise would have chosen abortion does not want to raise the baby. In addition, according to the definitions given in *Donum vitae*, surrogate motherhood necessarily involves IVF, and as was mentioned earlier partial ectogenesis does not. In sum, one can reject the permissibility of surrogate motherhood as understood in *Donum vitae* without rejecting the permissibility of using highly advanced incubators in lieu of abortion.

9.2.7 The Wrongful Experimentation Objection

The *wrongful experimentation* is perhaps the most powerful objection to partial ectogenesis. If scientific experimentation on human beings before birth is only permissible if directed to the healing or sustaining of the well-being of the individual not yet born, then to attempt partial ectogenesis would be wrong. The use of artificial wombs in lieu of abortion subjects the human fetus to risks, not for the sake of the human fetus's own welfare, but for the sake of the mother being free from pregnancy. Although, some day, techniques of partial ectogenesis may be made routine and no more risky than normal pregnancy, but all early attempts at partial ectogenesis would be wrongful experimentation.

However, as others have pointed out, ectogenesis could be developed naturally as an extension of saving premature babies. Experimental procedures undertaken to save the life of premature infants are fully acceptable given the principles suggested by John Paul II, since they would be directed towards the individual survival of the human beings in question. If these techniques were improved over time by means of this acceptable experimentation, the sustaining of very young human fetuses outside the womb would no longer be experimental but a common procedure subjecting its human subjects to no disproportionate risks. Partial ectogenesis may someday become *less risky* than normal gestation, since an artificial womb, presumably, would not get into car crashes, slip and fall, or be assaulted. Accepting that experimentation should only be undertaken for the good of the one experimented upon does not exclude the legitimate development of artificial wombs, if these artificial wombs are developed in the process of trying to save premature infants who would otherwise die. For the many couples experiencing painful premature deliveries due to an incompetent uterus, such technology would be a great blessing.

9.2.8 The Objection from the Right of a Child to Develop in the Womb of the Mother

One passage from John Paul II would seem to close the door entirely to partial ectogenesis. "Among the most important of these rights, mention must be made of the right to life, an integral part of which is the right of the child to develop in the mother's womb from the moment of conception" (John Paul II 1991, section 47). If one accepts Catholic teaching, artificial wombs in lieu of abortion would seem to be excluded by this passage.

I'm not sure this conclusion is necessary. It is not evident from this passage, nor from anything else written by John Paul II that he had considered the possibility of artificial wombs as a way of overcoming the impasse over abortion, let alone that he had considered and rejected this possibility. So, to apply this passage as if he had this question in mind is unjustified. In addition, the passage should not and would not be taken as a condemnation of inducement of labor, say a few days after or before the due date. But in the situation imagined, use of artificial wombs is not more dangerous to mother or child than inducements of labor which are now common and widely accepted by Catholic hospitals. Finally, one can grant the right of a child to develop in the womb from conception without also saying that this right extends through all nine months of pregnancy. Artificial wombs would not violate this right so long as the health of both mother and child is not endangered.

Doubtless there are objections and sources that could be brought to bear on this question that could lead to a different conclusion. However, even if it were morally impermissible to use highly advanced incubators in place of abortion, partial ectogenesis still might be counseled as the lesser of two evils in situations where a woman is determined to end her pregnancy. In cases in which an agent is determined to do wrong, it is permissible to counsel him or her to do the lesser of two evils (Finnis 1991, p. 98). If an agent is intent on harming an innocent person as an act of "revenge," and will not be deterred despite one's best efforts, one can counsel the agent to do less harm rather than more. When comparing abortion to the use of artificial wombs, an extermination to an extraction, it is clear that abortion involves a more serious evil, since abortion involves a more serious harm to the preborn, the intentional taking of human life, and partial ectogenesis, even if morally problematic, does not involve harms that are as serious. Thus, even if artificial wombs are morally impermissible considered in themselves, their use might still be urged in lieu of abortion, if a woman was determined to terminate her pregnancy in one way or another as it seems is often the case.

Thus far, I have sought to remove reasonable, but ultimately I believe mistaken, objections to partial ectogenesis. I have not addressed the positive case for limited use of partial ectogenesis. The most obvious answer is that artificial wombs could save innocent human life. There are approximately 43 million abortions each year in the world and between 1.2 and 1.6 million per year in the United States alone. If only a small percentage of abortions were eliminated by using artificial wombs, this would be a great service to the human community. Like orphanages and adoptions supported by virtually everyone, support of highly advanced incubators would help preserve the well-being of innocent preborn human persons who otherwise would be lost.

Artificial wombs could also be a great aid in helping couples facing infertility problems. Even aside from the abortion issue, such advanced incubators could help married couples who repeatedly lose pregnancies prior to natural viability because of maternal health problems, various kinds of maternal–fetal incompatibility, or other pathology. Imagine, a woman whose uterus had to be removed because of cancer could have an artificial womb constructed from those cancer free sections of her own uterine lining and then have this artificial uterus transplanted in her body facilitating "normal" conception, gestation, and birth. If an artificial womb may permissibly be used within a woman's body, it is difficult to see why it may not permissibly be used outside a woman's body.

Additionally, while some people allege that objections to abortion arise from an explicit or implicit desire to subjugate women by "tying them down" to children and pregnancy, in fact opposition to abortion arises from an affirmation of the equality and dignity of every single human being male or female, born or preborn. Support for partial ectogenesis in lieu of abortion would make this crystal clear to all. It is care and concern for the well-being of all human beings that lead to a condemnation of abortion, and the same care and concern lead to the approval of highly advanced incubators in lieu of abortion. There is no denying that the foreseen effects of giving live birth in cases of crisis pregnancy are characteristically much more difficult for the women involved than for the men. Not choosing abortion may be quite challenging, calling those involved to heroic generosity. Efforts should be made to lessen the difficulties borne uniquely by women in such crisis pregnancy situations through offering homes for mothers in need, providing child care, and making available other material and spiritual assistance. For example, many Catholic dioceses in the United States offer virtually full support of any woman facing a crisis pregnancy. Support of partial ectogenesis would be an extension of these efforts to make less difficult the burdens placed uniquely on pregnant women.

Imagine that scientists had discovered an injection that sped up the time of gestation? Rather than a full nine months of pregnancy, a woman who received this injection would give birth to a full term, perfectly healthy baby just nine minutes later. Imagine further that the injection was no more risky for mothers and their babies than normal gestation and childbirth. Would use of such injections be acceptable and welcomed to critics of abortion?

I believe that the answer would be yes. Although these injections would not be "natural," they would be no more contrary to nature, and wrong in a moral sense, than pain medication to ease the agony of labor. Rather than enduring morning sickness, interruption of educational or work schedules, and other hardships associated with a full nine months of pregnancy, women would be able to forego these difficulties, if they choose, without endangering the well-being of the child in question. Women who might otherwise be tempted to choose abortion rather than adoption (due to the long months of bonding with the child making adoption later extremely difficult) would be able to place their baby with a family before extensive bonding developed. Many who turn to abortion out of shame and fear of condemnation by others could speed up the gestation and deliver before anyone found out. Victims of rape impregnated by their attackers would not have to be reminded for nine months of their sexual assault. If such an injection existed, many women would be helped; many children preserved. All these considerations apply equally well to the use of artificial wombs as an alternative to abortion.

In the minds of many, and I count myself no exclusion, the phrase "artificial wombs" conjure images of Huxley's *Brave New World* or scenes from *Star Wars: Attack of the Clones*. I think of bizarre technology put to evil use. However, what we are talking about is no more ominous, bizarre, or evil than highly advanced versions of the NICUs widely used today to save the lives of thousands of premature infants. Like any technology, one can imagine the possibility of abuses, but the same thing is true of very primitive technologies such as fire and knives. Each year nearly half a million babies, more than 10% of births, take place at 36 weeks or before in the United States alone. Although caring for these children is currently very expensive and many of them become seriously disabled, we can hope that these drawbacks might be lessened or eliminated in the future. In other words, we have primitive artificial wombs and stone-age partial ectogenesis right now—and they are accepted by everyone. The use of technologically advanced incubators in lieu of abortion is therefore morally permissible, especially when the other likely alternative ends with a dead child and a wounded woman.

I do not wish to defend the view that artificial wombs may be used for any reason whatsoever but rather the more modest point that in situations in which a woman would otherwise have an abortion they would be permissible. The detailing of circumstances in which early birth making use of artificial wombs would be permissible falls outside the scope of my discussion. It may be, as mentioned earlier, that although the use of artificial wombs is not intrinsically evil that their use should be limited to relatively restricted circumstances, much as adoption now is not intrinsically evil but not permissible for frivolous reasons.

9.3 An End to the Abortion Debate?

Important public debates do not end when there is not a single person left on a given side of an issue, but rather when the vast majority of both sides come to a consensus. As noted in the first section of this chapter, the vast majority of defenders of abortion who have written about the topic in scholarly journals or books do not defend a right of extermination but rather the right of extraction. The termination of pregnancy and not the termination of human life is their stated goal. If they are consistent with what they have written, it would seem that the vast majority of these people could accept the use of artificial wombs in lieu of abortion. In the next section, it is argued that the artificial wombs in lieu of abortion could be accepted by many critics of abortion who have strong reason to support their use. If this is correct, then both ardent defenders and ardent critics of abortion could accept the permissibility of using artificial wombs in lieu of abortion. Of course, in this chapter, I have considered only a relatively small aspect of the "abortion debate," namely the intellectual debate, without taking into consideration the social, legal, and political aspects of the debate. Even if artificial wombs could placate the "intellectuals" on both sides of the matter, whether the use of artificial uteruses instead of abortion would also satisfy what Alasdair MacIntyre has called "plain persons" is a different matter. Nevertheless, although many scientific, social, legal, and economic hurdles remain, the day may come when, thanks to the use of artificial wombs, the abortion debate is as settled and distant as debates over slavery are today. In the meantime, I hope this book is a small step in the opposite direction, towards more debate, discussion, and dialogue about one of the most important and controversial issues of our time.

Bibliography

ACOG, American College of Obstetricians and Gynecologists, Committee on Ethics (1996). Sex selection. ACOG Committee Opinion No. 177. Washington, DC: ACOG, November.

ACOG, American College of Obstetricians and Gynecologists Executive Board (1997). Statement on intact dilatation and extraction. Retrieved from www. sdhealthyfamilies.org/media/pdf/ACOGAbortionPolicy.pdf (accessed June 8, 2010).

ACOG, American College of Obstetricians and Gynecologists Committee on Ethics (2007). The Limits of Conscientious Refusal in Reproductive Medicine: Opinion 385. Retrieved from www.acog.org/from_home/publications/ethics/co385.pdf (accessed June 8, 2010).

ACOG, American College of Obstetricians and Gynecologists Committee on Ethics (2007). Ethical Decision Making in Obstetrics and Gynecology: Opinion Number 390. Retrieved from www.acog.org/from_home/publications/ethics/co390.pdf (accessed June 8, 2010).

Akerlof, George, Yellen, Janet, & Katz, Michael (1996). An Analysis of Out-of-Wedlock Childbearing in the United States. *Quarterly Journal of Economics, 111*(2), 277–317.

Alcorn, Randy (2000). *Prolife Answers to Prochoice Arguments* (Expanded and Updated ed.). Portland: Multnomah Publishers.

Alexander, Greg R., Kogan, Michael, Bader, Deren, Carlo, Wally, Allen, Marilee, & Mor, Joanne (2003). US Birth Weight/Gestational Age-Specific Neonatal Mortality: 1995–1997 Rates for Whites, Hispanics, and Blacks. [Peer Reviewed]. *Pediatrics, 111*(1), 61–66.

Ali, Lorraine & Kelley, Raina (2008). The Curious Lives of Surrogates. *Newsweek*, April 7.

Anderson, Elizabeth (2004). Animal Rights and the Values of Nonhuman Life. In Cass R. Sunstein & Martha Nussbaum (Eds.), *Animal Rights: Current Debates and New Directions* (pp. 277–298). Oxford: Oxford University Press.

Anscombe, G. E. M. (1965). Contraception and Natural Law. *New Blackfriars, 46*, 517–521.

Anscombe, G. E. M. (1975). *Contraception and Chastity*. London: Catholic Truth Society.

Arey, Leslie Brainerd (1974). *Developmental Anatomy* (7th ed.). Philadelphia: Saunders.

Aristotle (1984). *The Complete Works of Aristotle.* Princeton: Princeton University Press.

Ashley, Benedict & Moraczewski, Albert (2001). Cloning, Aquinas, and the Embryonic Person. *National Catholic Bioethics Quarterly, 1*(2), 189–201.

Aulisio, Mark P. (1996). On the Importance of the Intention/Foresight Distinction. *American Catholic Philosophical Quarterly, 70*(2), 189–205.

Austriaco, Nicanor Pier Giorgio (2006). How to Navigate Species Boundaries: A Reply to The American Journal of Bioethics. *The National Catholic Bioethics Quarterly, 6*(1), 61–71.

Avila, David (2001). The Present Standing of the Human Embryo in U.S. Law. *National Catholic Bioethics Quarterly, 1*(2), 203–226.

Beckwith, Francis (2006). Defending Abortion Philosophically: A Review of David Boonin's *A Defense of Abortion. Journal of Medicine and Philosophy, 31,* 177–203.

Beckwith, Francis (2007). *Defending Life: A Moral and Legal Case Against Abortion Choice.* New York: Cambridge University Press.

Bermudez, Jose Luis (1996). The Moral Significance of Birth. *Ethics, 106*(2), 378–403.

Bhattacharyya, Swasti (2006). *Magical Progeny, Modern Technology: A Hindu Bioethics of Assisted Reproductive Technology.* New York: State University of New York Press.

Bitler, Marianne & Zavodny, Madeleine (2002). Did Abortion Legalization Reduce the Number of Unwanted Children? Evidence from Adoptions. *Perspectives on Sexual Reproductive Health, 34*(1), 25–33.

Boonin, David (2003). *A Defense of Abortion.* Cambridge, UK; New York: Cambridge University Press.

Boyle Jr., Joseph M. (1981). Human Action, Natural Rhythms, and Contraception: A Response to Noonan. *American Journal of Jurisprudence, 26*(1), 32–46.

Brody, Baruch (1975). *Abortion and the Sanctity of Human Life: A Philosophical View.* Cambridge: MIT Press.

Budziszewski, J. (2002). The Second Tablet Project. *First Things, 124,* 23–31.

Canavan, Francis (1994). Killing Abortionists: A Symposium. *First Things, 48,* 24–31. Retrieved from www.firstthings.com/article.php3?id_article=4524# Canavan (accessed May 28, 2010).

Cannold, Leslie (2000). *The Abortion Myth: Feminism, Morality, and the Hard Choices Women Make.* Hanover: University Press of England.

Card, Robert F. (2000). Infanticide and the Liberal View on Abortion. *Bioethics, 14*(4), 340–351.

Cavanaugh, Thomas (1996). The Intended/Foreseen Distinction's Ethical Relevance. *Philosophical Papers, 25*(3), 179–188.

CDF, Congregation for the Doctrine of the Faith (1987). *Donum Vitae: Instruction on Respect for Human Life in its Origins and on the Dignity of Procreation Replies to Certain Questions of the Day.* Vatican City.

Cioffi, Alfred (2001). Scientific Integrity. *National Catholic Bioethics Quarterly, 1*(2), 132.

Clark, R. M. & Chua, T. (1989). Breast Cancer and Pregnancy: The Ultimate Challenge. *Clinical Oncology, 1*(1), 11–18.

Clarke, W. N. (1995). *Explorations in Metaphysics.* Notre Dame: University of Notre Dame Press.

Cochrane, Linda (1996). *Forgiven and Set Free: A Post-Abortion Bible Study.* Grand Rapids, MI: Baker Books.

Coleman, Stephen (2004). *The Ethics of Artificial Uteruses: Implications for Reproduction and Abortion.* Hants: Ashgate Publishing.

Condic, Maureen L. (2003). Life: Defining the Beginning by the End. *First Things* (133), 50–54.

Crawford, Douglas & Mannion, Michael (1989). *Psycho-Spiritual Healing After an Abortion.* Kansas City, MO: Sheed & Ward.

Curtiss, Susan (1977). *Genie: A Psycholinguistic Study of a Modern Day "Wild Child".* New York: Academic Press.

Damschen, Gregor, Gomez-Lobo, Alfonso, & Schonecker, Dieter (2006). Sixteen Days? A Reply to B. Smith and B. Brogaard on the Beginning of Human Individuals. *Journal of Medicine and Philosophy, 31*(2), 165–175.

Davidson, Donald (1984). *Truth and Interpretation.* Oxford: Clarendon Press.

Derrida, Jacques (1973). *Speech and Phenomena* (David B. Allison, Trans.). Evanston: Northwestern University Press.

Diamond, E. (1999). Moral and Medical Considerations in the Management of Extrauterine Pregnancy. *Linacre Quarterly, 65,* 5–45.

Doerflinger, Richard (2002). Ditching Religion and Reality. *American Journal of Bioethics, 2*(1), 31–32.

Donagan, Alan (1977). *A Theory of Morality.* Chicago: University of Chicago Press.

Donceel, Joseph (1970). Immediate Animation and Delayed Hominization. *Theological Studies, 31*(1), 76–105.

Dworkin, Ronald (1994). *Life's Dominion: An Argument About Abortion, Euthanasia, and Individual Freedom.* New York: Vintage.

Dytrych, Zdenek, Matejček, Zdenek, Schüller, Vratislav, Friedman, David, & Friedman, Herbert L. (1975). Children Born to Women Denied Abortion. *Family Planning Perspectives, 7*(4), 165–171.

Engelhardt, H. Tristram (2000). The Sanctity of Life and the Concept of a Person. In Louis P. Pojman (Ed.), *Life and Death: A Reader in Moral Problems* (pp. 77–83). Belmont, CA: Wadsworth Publishing Co.

English, Jane (1975). Abortion and the Concept of a Person. *Canadian Journal of Philosophy, 5*(2), 233–243.

Epstein, Richard (2004). Animals as Objects, or Subjects, of Rights. In Cass R. Sunstein & Martha Nussbaum (Eds.), *Animal Rights: Current Debates and New Directions.* Oxford: Oxford University Press.

Esparza, Christina (2002). Infant's Body Found in Trash. *The Los Angeles Times,* July 10.

Feser, Edward (2005). Personal Identity and Self-Ownership. In Ellen Frankel Paul, Fred D. Miller & Jeffrey Paul (Eds.), *Personal Identity* (pp. 100–125). Cambridge: Cambridge University Press.

Finnis, John (1991). *Moral Absolutes: Tradition, Revision, and Truth.* Washington, DC: The Catholic University of American Press.

Finnis, John, Grisez, Germain, & Boyle, Joseph (2001). "Direct" and "Indirect": A Reply to Critics of our Action Theory. *The Thomist, 65*(1), 1–44.

Fischer, John Martin, Ravizza, Mark, & Copp, David (1993). Quinn on Double Effect: The Problem of "Closeness". *Ethics, 103*(4), 707–725.

Ford, Norman (1988). *When Did I Begin? Conception of the Human Individual in History, Philosophy and Science.* Cambridge: Cambridge University Press.

Francione, Gary (2004). Animals—Property or Person? In Cass R. Sunstein & Martha Nussbaum (Eds.), *Animal Rights: Current Debates and New Directions* (pp. 108–142). Oxford: Oxford University Press.

George, Robert P. (1994). Killing Abortionists: A Symposium. *First Things*, (48), 24–31.

George, Robert P. (2001). *The Clash of Orthodoxies: Law, Religion, and Morality in Crisis.* Wilmington, DE: ISI Press.

George, Robert P. & Lee, Patrick (2005). Acorns and Embryos. *The New Atlantis*, 2(7), 90–100.

George, Robert P. & Tollefsen, Christopher (2008a). *Embryo: A Defense of Human Life.* New York: Doubleday.

George, Robert P. & Tollefsen, Christopher (2008b). Embryonic Debate: A Reply to William Saletan, Liberal Bioethics Writer, Former Embryo. *National Review Online.* Retrieved from http://article.nationalreview.com/?q=Y2IxM2QzNDc4OTJhNmJjODEzMDBiYjRiZjQyOTg3YWM (accessed June 8, 2010).

Gewirth, Alan (1978). *Reason and Morality.* Chicago: University of Chicago Press.

Gissler, Mika, Hemminki, Elina, & Lonnqvist, Jouko (1996). Suicides after pregnancy in Finland, 1987–94: register linkage study. *British Medical Journal*, 313, 1341–1344.

Gleason, Gerald (1999). Is the Medical Management of Ectopic Pregnancy by the Administration of Methotrexate Morally Acceptable? In Luke Gormally (Ed.), *Issues for a Catholic Bioethic.* London: Linacre Center.

Gomez-Lobo, Alfonso (2007). Individuality and Human Beginnings: A Reply to David DeGrazia. *The Journal of Law, Medicine & Ethics*, 35(3), 457–462.

Grall, Timothy (2005). *Support Providers 2002.* from www.census.gov/prod/2005pubs/p70–99.pdf (accessed June 8, 2010).

Grey, Ronald H. & Wu, Ling Yu (2000). Subfertility and Risk of Spontaneous Abortion. *American Journal of Public Health*, 90(9), 1452–1454.

Green, Ronald (2001). *The Human Embryo Research Debates: Bioethics in the Vortex of Controversy.* Oxford: Oxford University.

Green, Ronald (2002). Determining Moral Status. *American Journal of Bioethics*, 2(1), 20–30.

Grisez, Germain (1964). *Contraception and the Natural Law.* Milwaukee, WI: The Bruce Publishing Company.

Grisez, Germain (1970). Toward a Consistent Natural Law Ethics of Killing. *American Journal of Jurisprudence*, 15, 64–96.

Haldane, John (2008). Recognizing Humanity. *Journal of Applied Philosophy*, 25(4), 301–313.

Haldane, John & Lee, Patrick (2003). Aquinas on Human Ensoulment, Abortion and the Value of Life. *Philosophy*, 78(2), 255–278.

Hallett, Garth L. & Kaczor, Christopher (1995). Greater Good: The Case for Proportionalism. *Review of Metaphysics*, 50(4), 898–899.

Harman, Elizabeth (2000). Creation Ethics: The Moral Status of Early Fetuses and the Ethics of Abortion. *Philosophy and Public Affairs*, 28(4), 310–324.

Harman, Elizabeth (2007). How is the Ethics of Stem Cell Research Different from the Ethics of Abortion? *Metaphilosophy, 38*(2–3), 207–225.

Harris, John (1999). The Concept of the Person and the Value of Life. *Kennedy Institute of Ethics Journal, 9*(4), 293–308.

Harris, John & Holm, Soren (2003). Abortion. In Hugh LaFollette (Ed.), *The Oxford Handbook of Practical Ethics* (pp. 112–135). Oxford: Oxford University Press.

Harter, Thomas (2008). Overcoming the Organ Shortage: Failing Means and Radical Reform. *HEC Forum: An Interdisciplinary Journal on Hospitals' Ethical and Legal Issues, 20*(2), 155–182.

Hassoun, Nicole & Kriegel, Uriah (2008). Consciousness and the Moral Permissibility of Infanticide. *Journal of Applied Philosophy, 25*(1), 45–55.

Hendin, Herbert (1998). *Seduced by Death: Doctors, Patients and Assisted Suicide* (Revised and Updated). New York: W. W. Norton & Company.

Hershenov, David (2005). Persons as Proper Parts of Organisms. *Theoria, 71*(1), 29–37.

Hershenov, David B. (2008). A Hylomorphic Account of Thought Experiments Concerning Personal Identity. *American Catholic Philosophical Quarterly, 82*(3), 481–502.

Hitchens, Christopher (2003). Fetal Distraction. *Vanity Fair* (February), 84–88.

Hoche, Alfred & Binding, Karl (1920). *Die Freigabe der Vernichtung Lebensunwertem Lebens.* Leipzig: Felix Meiner Verlag.

Hoopes, Tom (2002). When Abortion Kills Twice: The Breast-Cancer Link. *Crisis, 20*(8), 20–25.

Hopson, Janet (1998). Fetal Psychology. *Psychology Today, 31*(5), 44–49.

Hursthouse, Rosalind (1987). *Beginning Lives.* Oxford: Oxford University Press.

Hursthouse, Rosalind (1991). Virtue Theory and Abortion. *Philosophy and Public Affairs, 20*(3), 223–246.

James, David N. (1987). Ectogenesis: A Reply to Singer and Well's 'The Reproductive Revolution' and 'Making Babies.' *Bioethics, 1*(1), 80–89.

Jansson, Bengt (1965). Mental Disorders After Abortion. *Acta Psychiatrica Scandinavica, 41*, 87–110.

John Paul II, Pope (1991). *Centesimus annus.* Vatican City: Vatican.

Johnson, Mark (2002). The Moral Status of Embryonic Human Life. In Edward J. Furton & Louise A. Mitchell (Eds.), *What is Man, O Lord?: The Human Person in a Biotech Age: Eighteenth Workshop for Bishops* (pp. 181–198). Boston: National Catholic Bioethics Center.

Jones, David Albert (2005). *The Soul of the Embryo: An Enquiry into the Status of the Human Embryo in the Christian Tradition.* London: Continuum.

Kaczor, Christopher (2002). *Proportionalism and the Natural Law Tradition.* Washington DC: The Catholic University of America Press.

Kaczor, Christopher (2005). *The Edge of Life: Human Dignity and Contemporary Bioethics.* Dordrecht: Springer.

Kaczor, Christopher (2009). The Ethics of Ectopic Pregnancy: A Critical Reconsideration of Salpingostomy and Methotrexate. *Linacre Quarterly: A Journal of the Philosophy and Ethics of Medical Practice, 76*(3), 265–282.

Kain, Patrick (2009). Kant's Defense of Human Moral Status. *Journal of the History of Philosophy 47*(1), 59–101.

236 Bibliography

Kamm, Francis (1992). *Creation and Abortion: A Study in Moral and Legal Philosophy*. Oxford: Oxford University Press.

Kane, Thomas & Staiger, Douglas (1996). Teen Motherhood and Abortion Access. *Quarterly Journal of Economics, 111*(2), 467–506.

Kant, Immanuel (1993). *Grounding for the Metaphysics of Morals* (James E. Ellington, Trans.). Indianapolis: Hackett Publishers.

Kavanaugh, John (2001). *Who Count as Persons? Human Identity and the Ethics of Killing*. Washington, DC: Georgetown University Press.

Keown, John (2002). *Euthanasia, Ethics and Public Policy: An Argument Against Legalisation*. Cambridge: Cambridge University Press.

Kirton, Isabella (1998). *Spirit Child: Healing the Wound of Abortion*. Forres: Findhorn Press.

Kluger-Bell, Kim (1998). *Unspeakable Losses: Understanding the Experience of Pregnancy Loss, Miscarriage and Abortion*. New York: W. W. Norton & Company.

Korfmacher, Carsten (2006). Personal Identity. *The Internet Encyclopedia of Philosophy*. Retrieved from www.utm.edu/RESEARCH/IEP/p/person-i.htm (accessed June 8, 2010).

Kushner, Eve (1998). *Experiencing Abortion: A Weaving of Women's Words*. New York: Haworth Park Press.

Larsen, William J. (1993). *Human Embryology*. New York: Churchill Livingstone.

Lee, Patrick (1996). *Abortion and Unborn Human Life*. Washington, DC: The Catholic University of America Press.

Lee, Patrick (1998). Human Beings are Animals. In Robert P. George (Ed.), *Natural Law and Moral Inquiry: Ethics, Metaphysics, and Politics in the Work of Germain Grisez*. Washington, DC: Georgetown University Press.

Lee, Patrick & George, Robert P. (2007). *Body–Self Dualism in Contemporary Ethics and Politics*. New York: Cambridge University Press.

Levinas, Emmanuel (1980). *Totality and Infinity: An Essay on Exteriority* (4th ed.). Dordrecht: Springer.

Levine, Phillip, Staiger, Douglas, Kane, Thomas, & Zimmerman, David (1999). *Roe v. Wade* and American Fertility. *American Journal of Public Health, 89*(2), 199–203.

Liao, S. Matthew (2006a). The Embryo Rescue Case. *Theoretical Medicine and Bioethics, 27*(2), 141–147.

Liao, S. Matthew (2006b). The Organism View Defended. *Monist, 89*(3), 334–350.

Liao, S. Matthew (2010a). The Basis of Human Moral Status. *Journal of Moral Philosophy, 7*(2), 159–179.

Liao, S. Matthew (2010b). Twinning, Inorganic Replacement, and the Organism View. *Ratio, 23*(1), 59–72.

Lindemann, Hilde & Verkerk, Marian (2008). Ending the Life of a Newborn: The Groningen Protocol. *The Hastings Center Report, 38*(1), 42–51.

Little, Margaret Olivia (2003). Abortion. In R. G. Frey & Christopher Heath Wellman (Eds.), *A Companion to Applied Ethics*. Malden, MA: Blackwell Publishing.

Little, Margaret Olivia (2005). The Moral Permissibility of Abortion. In Andrew

I. Cohen & Christopher Heath Wellman (Eds.), *Contemporary Debates in Applied Ethics* (pp. 27–39). Oxford: Blackwell Publishing.

Locke, John (1996). *An Essay Concerning Human Understanding.* Indianapolis: Hackett.

Lorenz, J. M. (2001). The Outcome of Extreme Prematurity. *Seminars in Perinatology, 25*(5), 348–359.

MacIntyre, Alasdair (1992). Utilitarianism and the Presuppositions of Cost–Benefit Analysis. In John Martin Gilroy & Maurice Wade (Eds.), *The Moral Dimensions of Public Policy Choice: Beyond the Market Paradigm* (pp. 179–194). Pittsburgh: University of Pittsburgh Press.

MacIntyre, Alasdair (1999). *Dependent Rational Animals: Why Human Beings Need the Virtues.* Chicago: Open Court.

Maestri, William (2000). *Do Not Lose Hope: Healing the Wounded Heart of Women Who Have Had Abortions.* New York: Alba House.

Malcolm, Norman (1977). *Thought and Knowledge.* Ithaca: Cornell University Press.

Marquis, Donald (1991). Four Versions of Double Effect. *Journal of Medicine and Philosophy, 16*(5), 515–544.

Marquis, Donald (1999). Why Abortion is Immoral. In Helga Kuhse & Peter Singer (Eds.), *Bioethics: An Anthology.* Malden, MA: Blackwell Publishing.

Marquis, Donald (2007). Abortion Revisited. In Bonnie Steinbock (Ed.), *The Oxford Handbook of Bioethics.* Oxford: Oxford University Press, pp. 395–415.

Massé, Synda & Phillips, Joan (1998). *Her Choice to Heal: Finding Spiritual and Emotional Peace After Abortion.* Colorado Springs, CO: Chariot Victor Publishing.

Mathewes-Green, Frederica (1997). *Real Choices: Listening to Women; Looking for Alternatives to Abortion.* Ben Lomond, CA: Conciliar Press.

May, William (1998). Methotrexate and Ectopic Pregnancy. *Ethics and Medics, 23*(3), 1–2.

McCormick, Richard (1991). Who or What Is the Preembryo? *Kennedy Institute of Ethics Journal, 1*(1), 1–15.

McCullough, David (2001). *John Adams.* New York: Simon & Schuster.

McDonagh, Eileen (1996). *Breaking the Abortion Deadlock: From Choice to Consent.* Oxford: Oxford University Press.

McMahan, Jeff (2002). *The Ethics of Killing: Problems at the Margins of Life.* Oxford: Oxford University Press.

McMahan, Jeff (2003). Animals. In R. G. Frey & Christopher Heath Wellman (Eds.), *A Companion to Applied Ethics.* Malden, MA: Blackwell Publishing.

McMahan, Jeff (2005). Summary of *The Ethics of Killing: Problems at the Margins of Life. Philosophical Books, 46*(1), 1–3.

McMahan, Jeff (2007). Infanticide. *Utilitas, 19*(2), 1–29.

McMahan, Jeff (2008). Challenges To Human Equality. *The Journal of Ethics, 12*(1), 81–104

Miller, Franklin G. & Truog, Robert D. (2009). The Incoherence of Determining Death by Neurological Criteria: A Commentary on *Controversies in the Determination of Death*, A White Paper by the President's Council on Bioethics. *Kennedy Institute of Ethics Journal, 19*(2), 185–193.

Milliez, J. M. (2007). Sex Selection for Non-Medical Purposes. *Reproductive BioMedicine Online, 14*, 114–117.

Modvig, Jens, Schmidt, Lone, & Damsgaard, Mogens T. (1990). Measurement of Total Risk of Spontaneous Abortion: The Virtue of Conditional Risk Estimation. *American Journal of Epidemiology, 132*(6), 1021–1037.

Moore, Keith L. (1987). *Before We Are Born* (2nd ed.), Washington DC: Carnegie Institution of Washington.

Moraczewski, Albert (1996a). Managing Tubal Pregnancies: Part 1. *Ethics & Medics, 21*(6), 1–3.

Moraczewski, Albert (1996b). Managing Tubal Pregnancies: Part 2. *Ethics & Medics, 21*(8), 3–4.

Morgan, Christopher L., Evans, Marc, Peters, John R., & Currie, Craig (1997). Mental Health may Deteriorate as a Direct Effect of Induced Abortion. *British Medical Journal, 314*, 902.

Morowitz, Harold J. & Terfil, James S. (1992). *The Facts of Life: Science and the Abortion Controversy*. Oxford: Oxford University Press.

Najman, J. M., Morrison, J., Williams, G., Andersen, M., & Keeping, J. D. (1991). The Mental Health of Women 6 Months After They Give Birth to an Unwanted Baby: A Longitudinal Study. *Social Science & Medicine, 32*(3), 214–247.

Napier, Stephen (2008). Twinning, Substance, and Identity through Time: A Reply to McMahan. *National Catholic Bioethics Quarterly, 8*(2), 255–264.

Nathanson, Bernard N. (2001). *The Hand of God: A Journey from Death to Life by the Abortion Doctor Who Changed His Mind*. Washington, DC: Regnery Pub.

Nathanson, Bernard N. with Ostling, Richard N. (1979). *Aborting America*. Toronto: Life Cycle Books.

National Academy of Sciences (2005). *Guidelines for Human Embryonic Stem Cell Research*. Washington, DC: The National Academies Press.

Nobbs, Christopher (2007). Probability Potentiality. *Cambridge Quarterly of Healthcare Ethics, 16*, 204–247.

Noonan, John (1970). An Almost Absolute Value in History. In [Reprint] Ronald Munson (Ed.), *Intervention and Reflection: Basic Issues in Medical Ethics* (5th ed., pp. 66–69). Belmont, CA: Wadsworth Publishing Co. 1996.

Noonan, John (1981). The Experience of Pain by the Unborn. In Thomas Hilgers, Dennis Horan & David D. Mall (Eds.), *New Perspectives on Human Abortion*. Frederick, MD: University Publications of America.

Nussbaum, Martha (2004). Beyond Compassion and Humanity: Justice for Non-Human Animals. In Cass R. Sunstein & Martha Nussbaum (Eds.), *Animal Rights: Current Debates and New Directions* (pp. 299–320). Oxford: Oxford University Press.

Nussbaum, Martha (2006). *Frontiers of Justice: Disability, Nationality, Species Membership*. Cambridge, MA: The Belknap Press.

Nussbaum, Martha (2008). Hiding From Humanity: Replies to Charlton, Haldane, Archard, and Brooks. *Journal of Applied Philosophy, 25*(4), 335–349.

Nykiel, Connie (1997). *No One Told Me I Could Cry*. Toronto: Life Cycle Books.

Obama, Barack (2008). *The Audacity of Hope: Thoughts on Reclaiming the American Dream*. New York: Vintage.

Oderberg, David (2000). *Applied Ethics: A Non-Consequentialist Approach*. Oxford: Blackwell Publishers.

Oderberg, David S. (2008). The Metaphysical Status of the Embryo: Some Arguments Revisited. *Journal of Applied Philosophy, 25*(4), 263–276.

Olson, Eric (1997a). *The Human Animal: Personal Identity Without Psychology*. New York: Oxford University Press.

Olson, Eric T. (1997b). Was I Ever a Fetus? *Philosophy and Phenomenological Research, 57*(1), 95–110.

Olson, Eric T. (2008). Personal Identity. *Stanford Encyclopedia of Philosophy*. Retrieved from http://plato.stanford.edu/entries/identity-personal/ (accessed June 8, 2010).

Parfit, Derek (1987). *Reasons and Persons*. New York: Oxford University Press.

Parker, Kathleen (2009). When Abortion Isn't a Choice. *Washington Post*. Retrieved from www.washingtonpost.com/wp-dyn/content/article/2009/11/10/AR2009111013891.html (accessed June 8, 2010).

Peach, Andrew (2007). Late- vs. Early Term Abortion: A Thomistic Analysis. *The Thomist, 71*(1), 113–141.

Piontelli, Alessandra (1992). *From Fetus to Child: An Observational and Psychoanalytic Study*. London: Routledge.

Plato (1971). *Gorgias* (Walter Hamilton, Trans.). New York: Penguin Books.

Pruss, Alexander (2008). Two Remarks on Thomson's Violinist Argument for Abortion, *Alexander Pruss's Blog* (Vol. 2010).

Purdy, Laura & Tooley, Michael (1974). Is Abortion Murder? In Robert Perkins (Ed.), *Abortion: Pro and Con* (pp. 129–149). Cambridge, MA: Schenkman Publishers.

Quinn, Warren (1989). Actions, Intentions, and Consequences: The Doctrine of Double Effect. *Philosophy and Public Affairs, 18*(4), 334–351.

Rachels, James (1975). Active and Passive Euthanasia. *New England Journal of Medicine, 292*(2), 78–80.

Reardon, David (1987). *Aborted Women: Silent No More*. Chicago: Loyola University Press.

Reardon, David (1996). *The Jericho Plan: Breaking Down the Walls which Prevent Post-Abortion Healing*. Springfield, IL: Acorn Books.

Reardon, David C., Cougle, Jesse R., Rue, Vincent M., Shuping, Martha W., Coleman, Priscilla K., & Ney, Philip G. (2003). Psychiatric Admissions of Low Income Women Following Abortion and Childbirth. *Canadian Medical Association Journal, 168*(10), 1253–1257.

Regan, Tom (1985). *The Case for Animal Rights*. Berkeley: University of California Press.

Reichmann, James (1985). *Philosophy of the Human Person*. Chicago: Loyola University Press.

Reichmann, James (2000). *Evolution, Animal 'Rights,' and the Environment*. Washington, DC: The Catholic University of America Press.

Reisser, Teri & Reisser, Paul (2000). *A Solitary Sorrow: Finding Healing and Wholeness After Abortion*. Wheaton, IL: H. Shaw Publishers.

Rifkin, Jeremy (2002). The End of Pregnancy: Within a Generation There Will Probably Be Mass Use of Artificial Wombs to Grow Babies. *The*

Guardian of London. Retrieved from www.guardian.co.uk/Archive/Article/ 0,4273,4337092,00.html (accessed June 8, 2010).

Ring-Cassidy, Elizabeth & Gentles, Ian (2002). *Women's Health after Abortion: The Medical and Psychological Evidence*. Toronto: de Veber Institute.

Rogers, Wendy, Ballantyne, Angela, & Draper, Heather (2007). Is Sex-Selective Abortion Morally Justified and Should It Be Prohibited? *Bioethics, 21*(9), 520–524.

Rubenfeld, Jed (1991). On the Legal Status of the Proposition that "Life Begins at Conception." *Stanford Law Review, 43*, 533–635.

Savulescu, Julian (2001). Is Current Practice Around Late Termination of Pregnancy Eugenic and Discriminatory? Maternal Interests and Abortion. *Journal of Medical Ethics, 27*(3), 165–171.

Savulescu, Julian (2002). Abortion, Embryo Destruction and the Future of Value Argument. *Journal of Medical Ethics, 25*(3), 133–135.

Schmutz, Stephanie D. (2002). Infanticide or Civil Rights for Women: Did the Supreme Court Go Too Far in *Stenberg v. Carhart? Houston Law Review, 39*, 530–566.

Schwarz, Stephen (1990). *The Moral Question of Abortion*. Chicago: Loyola University Press.

Sherwin, Susan (1996). Abortion Through a Feminist Ethics Lens. In Ronald Munson (Ed.), *Intervention and Reflection: Basic Issues in Medical Ethics* (5th ed.). Belmont, CA: Wadsworth Publishing Co.

Shettles, L. (1990). Tubal Embryo Successfully Transplanted in Utero. *American Journal of Obstetrics and Gynecology, 163*(6), 2026–2027.

Shewmon, D. Alan (1998). Brainstem Death, Brain Death, and Death: A Critical Re-Evaluation. *Issues in Law & Medicine, 14*(2), 125–145.

Shewmon, D. Alan (1999). Is it Reasonable to Use the UK Protocol for the Clinical Diagnosis of 'Brain Stem Death' as a Basis for Diagnosing Death? In Luke Gormally (Ed.), *Issues for a Catholic Bioethic*. London: Linacre Center.

Shewmon, D. Alan (2001). The Brain and Somatic Integration: Insights into the Standard Biological Rationale for Equating 'Brain Death' with Death. *Journal of Medicine and Philosophy, 26*(5), 475–478.

Shewmon, D. Alan (2004). The Dead Donor Rule: Lessons from Linguistics? *Kennedy Institute of Ethics Journal, 14*(3), 277–300.

Shewmon, D. Alan (2009). Brain Death: Can It Be Resuscitated? *Hastings Center Report, 39*(2), 18–24.

Singer, Peter (1979). *Practical Ethics*. Cambridge: Cambridge University Press.

Singer, Peter (1993). *Practical Ethics* (2nd ed.). Cambridge: Cambridge University Press.

Singer, Peter (1994). *Rethinking Life & Death: The Collapse of Our Traditional Ethics*. New York: St. Martin's Press.

Singer, Peter (2000). *Writings on an Ethical Life*. New York: Ecco Press.

Singer, Peter & Wells, Deane (1984). *The Reproduction Revolution: New Ways of Making Babies*. Oxford: Oxford University Press.

Smith, Janet (1991). *Humanae Vitae: A Generation Later*. Washington, DC: The Catholic University of America Press.

Smolin, David M. (2000). The Supreme Court 2000: A Symposium. *First Things*, (106), 27.

Spitzer, Robert (2000). *Healing the Culture: A Commonsense Philosophy of Happiness, Freedom, and Life Issues.* San Francisco: Ignatius Press.

Steinbock, Bonnie (1992). *Life before Birth: The Moral and Legal Status of Embryos and Fetuses.* New York: Oxford University Press.

Stich, Stephen (1983). *From Folk Psychology to Cognitive Science: The Case Against Belief.* Cambridge, MA: MIT Press.

Strahan, Thomas (2001). *Detrimental Effects of Abortion.* Springfield, IL: Acorn Books.

Stretton, Dean (2008). Critical Notice—Defending Life: A Moral and Legal Case Against Abortion Choice by Francis J. Beckwith. [review article]. *Journal of Medical Ethics, 34*(11), 793–797.

Sumner, L. W. (1981). *Abortion and Moral Theory.* Princeton: Princeton University Press.

Swope, Paul (1998). Abortion: A Failure to Communicate. *First Things,* (82), 31–35.

Taylor, Paul (1986). *Respect for Nature: A Theory of Environmental Ethics.* Princeton: Princeton University Press.

Thomson, Judith Jarvis (1971). A Defense of Abortion. *Philosophy and Public Affairs, 1*(1), 47–66.

Thomson, Judith Jarvis (1995). Abortion: Whose Right. *Boston Review, 20*(3), 11–15.

Tollefsen, Christopher (2008). The Ever-Conscious View: A Critique. *National Catholic Bioethics Quarterly 8*(1), 43–48.

Tooley, Michael (1972). Abortion and Infanticide. *Philosophy and Public Affairs, 2*(1) (Autumn), 37–65.

Tooley, Michael (1983). *Abortion and Infanticide.* Oxford: Oxford University Press.

Tooley, Michael, Wolf-Devine, Celia, Devine, Philip E., & Jaggar, Alison M. (2009). *Abortion: Three Perspectives.* New York: Oxford University Press.

Torre-Bueno, Ava (1997). *Peace After Abortion* (2nd ed.). San Diego, CA: Pimpernel Press.

Tribe, Laurence H. (1997). *Constitutional Analysis of "Partial Birth Abortion" Ban.* March 6. Available online at www.now.org/issues/abortion/dxanalysis. htm (accessed May 28, 2010).

United States Council of Catholic Bishops, USCCB (2001). *Ethical and Religious Directives for Catholic Health Care Services* (4th ed.). Washington DC: USCCB Publishing Services.

Varelius, Jukka (2009). Minimally Conscious State and Human Dignity. *Neuroethics, 2*(1), 35–50.

Warnock, Mary (1988). *A Question of Life: The Warnock Report on Human Fertilization and Embryology.* Oxford.

Warnock, Mary (2004). *An Intelligent Person's Guide to Ethics.* New York/ London: Overlook.

Warren, Mary Anne (1973). The Personhood Argument in Favor of Abortion. In [Reprint] Louis P. Pojman (Ed.), *Life and Death: A Reader in Moral Problems* (pp. 261–267). Belmont, CA: Wadsworth Publishing Co. 2000.

Warren, Mary Anne (1981). Do Potential Persons Have Rights? In Ernest Partridge (Ed.), *Responsibilities to Future Generations* (pp. 261–274). Buffalo, NY: Prometheus Books.

Warren, Mary Anne (1989). The Moral Significance of Birth. *Hypatia, 4*(3), 46–65.

Warren, Mary Anne (1996). On the Moral and Legal Status of Abortion. In Ronald Munson (Ed.), *Intervention and Reflection: Basic Issues in Medical Ethics* (5th ed.). Belmont, CA: Wadsworth Publishing Co. The article originally appeared in *The Monist, 57*(1) (1973), 43–61.

Warren, Mary Anne (1997). *Moral Status: Obligations to Persons and Other Living Things.* Oxford: Clarendon Press.

Warren, Mary Anne (1998). Abortion. In Helga Kuhse & Peter Singer (Eds.), *A Companion to Bioethics* (pp. 127–134). Oxford: Blackwell Publishers.

Warren, Mary Anne (1999). Sex Selection: Individual Choice or Cultural Coercion? In Helga Kuhse & Peter Singer (Eds.), *Bioethics: An Anthology* (pp. 137–142). Oxford: Blackwell Publishers.

Warren, Mary Anne (2000). The Moral Difference between Infanticide and Abortion: A Response to Robert Card. *Bioethics, 14*(4), 352–359.

Weaver, D. R. & Reppert, S. M. (1989). Direct in Utero Perception of Light by the Mammalian Fetus. *Brain Research: Developmental Brain Research, 47*(1), 151–155.

Werner, Richard (1973). Abortion: the Ontological and Moral Status of the Unborn. In Richard A. Wasserstrom (Ed.), *Today's Moral Problems* (2nd ed.) (pp. 51–73). New York: Macmillan.

Wertheimer, Roger (1971). Understanding the Abortion Argument. *Philosophy and Public Affairs, 1*(1), 67–95.

Wolf, Naomi (1995). Our Bodies, Our Souls. *The New Republic*, October 16.

Zilberberg, Julie (2007). Sex Selection and Restricting Abortion and Sex Determination. *Bioethics, 21*(9), 517–519.

Zimmerman, Sacha (2003). The Fetal Position: The Real Threat to *Roe v. Wade. The New Republic*, August 18.

Index